THAI MASSAGE MADE EASY

LEARN HOW TO DO THAI MASSAGE EVEN IF YOU HAVE NO EXPERIENCE

CÉSAR ARIEL SANDOVAL

CONTENTS

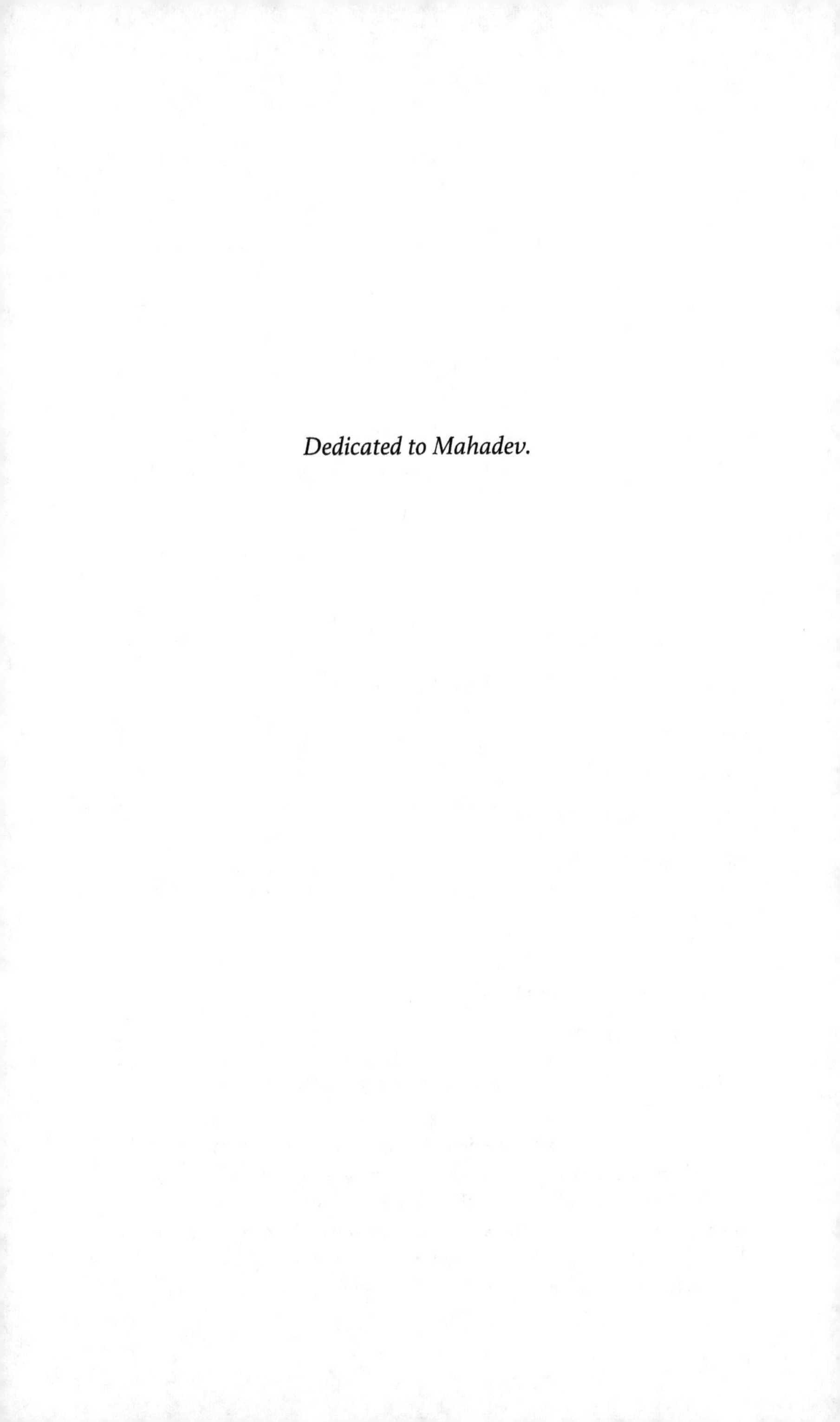

Dedicated to Mahadev.

A GIFT

If you want a perfect complement to what you'll see on the following pages, I recommend that you sign up for the videos that come with this book.

I have created this online course so that you have the opportunity to learn in a more enjoyable and efficient way, through step-by-step explanatory videos, as if you were by my side. I hope you find it useful.

Request access to the free online course by typing this url or by scanning the QR code:

https://learnthaimassage.net/videoguide

PROLOGUE

In March 2002 I decided to make a major change in my life. I dropped out college, where I was studying English translation, and started my journey to become a masseur. It was not that I no longer liked the career, but I felt suffocated, and I had other interests that were way more interesting to me than the idea of translating texts. My room was full of books on spirituality and natural therapies that I could not read, basically because university did not give me time for anything else. My heart was calling me more and more towards health and bodywork, and less and less to sitting in front of the computer all day. So I dropped out my university life, and with the extra time I started to read everything I could get my hands on, and I also started to learn and practice different massage techniques. In 2003 I found out about Thai massage and started doing it. I was impressed by its technical richness, by the way of involving different parts of the body in the therapy, and above all, by the idea of offering a completely different experience, both for the receiver and for the therapist. Thai massage transformed me into a more complete masseuse, it helped me stand out when I was working as a spa therapist on Royal Caribbean cruises, thanks to Thai massage I managed to learn to work with my body weight, to have a better posture, to improve my health while helping to restore the health of others. Today I want to share with you some of what I have learned over the years of practice and research in different schools and with different teachers in and out of Thailand. I have created this book so that you can learn the basics of therapeutic Thai massage, important concepts and techniques for you and the people you touch, so that you can give a good Thai session even if you have never done a massage before.

So, this book is for you if you are a therapist, if you work with some kind of body or energy therapy, and if you are looking to broaden your experience, add the knowledge of a traditional ethnic medicine. Also, this book is for you if you are a yoga teacher and you are interested in coupling a therapy that is closely related to yoga asanas.

You will like this book if you are a person who has never been involved in natural therapies, but you feel attracted to techniques that help to improve health in a natural way and you have a vocation of service.

I intend this book to be a starting point, a reference that encourages you to take your first steps and experience what Thai massage can do for you, and for others. I would love to help you discover the potential of Thai massage in your therapies and transform your treatments and your life, just as it did for me. And if you feel like going further and deeper, I can help you with my in-person courses in Barcelona, as well as with my online courses that you will find at learnthaimassage.net. May this be the beginning of something great for you.

· · ·

BEST REGARDS.

CÉSAR A. Sandoval

Founder of Shivathai https://shivathai.net & https://learn thaimassage.net

Girona, Spain

29/11/2018

~

NOTES **on the 2023 edition**

I THOUGHT it was time to revise the content of the book. In doing so, I discovered that there were some topics that I did not include in the first version, and that were important.

The first of these topics is a Thai massage adapted to a massage table. Although Thai massage is intended to be performed at ground level, I think it is useful to know what we can do on the massage table (and how) based on Thai massage. By doing so you will be able to improve on the techniques you are already using and achieve better results.

The second topic is a Thai massage with the feet. Working with your feet allows you to lower the amount of energy you use in your work. Your messaging becomes more exotic, clients love it, and you can work with even larger and heavier clients with little effort.

The third topic I have added to the book is a Thai abdominal massage. In my courses, when I do abdominal massages, I always ask who of the girls is having period pain. I do this because the following month I usually contact them to ask how they have been doing with their period pain, and in all cases the pain subsides either completely or partially. Abdominal massage is one of the most therapeutic things I know of because it influences the function of internal organs, energy, emotions, and the health of the lower back.

The fourth and last topic is Thai acupressure, although it is a more invasive technique, it usually gives very good results.

I have dedicated a chapter to each topic with simplified routines so that you can easily learn them and put them into practice right away.

I hope this update will push you one step closer to excellence.

BLESSINGS.

CESAR

TARRAGONA, April 11, 2023

PART I

TOPICS TO CONSIDER

Here I am going to cover some preliminary topics: you can skip these chapters and go directly to the practice part, but I advise you to spend some time on it in order to have a foundation for your own practice. When you understand the underlying foundation of this style, your style of massage changes as well.

CHAPTER 1
CONCEPTS AND MYTHS

Over the years I have met people who don't know what Thai massage is, people who think they know what it is, and practitioners who have a notion but don't know how to define it clearly. So in this section I am going to solve the common doubts and give some definitions.

Traditional Thai massage, also known as nuad boran, nuat boran, nuadborarn or thai yoga massage, is a physical therapy that uses different tools and techniques to heal the body, and, eventually, balance the energy of the recipient. I will briefly detail why this definition is so important.

It is a therapy because it is part of the 5 branches of traditional Thai medicine, namely: the external or ortho-pedic branch (here we find all the disciplines where the body is touched and / or manipulated, including massage), then there is the internal branch, divinatory sciences, shamanic medicine and Buddhism.

Many people think that Thai massage is just a combina-tion of acupressure and passive yoga, or simply a sequence of assisted stretches on the floor level. Thai massage as such employs different tools that can be integrated into a massage treatment depending on the knowledge and expertise of the practitioner. Thus, techniques such as acupressure and passive stretching are used in massage, but also chiropractic, kneading, friction, percussion, internal organ massage, etc. to heal the body. As an external therapy, massage is intended to treat a large number of pathologies affecting the body. This is where we must make a distinction between general massage (this is the type of Thai massage taught in most massage schools), which is intended to relax and mobilize the body, and therapeutic massage, which is used to treat different pathologies. The main difference is that general massage uses a generic routine for everyone, and therapeutic massage customizes the session according to the characteristics and needs of the receiver. Although the massage is designed to treat the physical body, according to Thai medicine, every problem arises from an imbalance in the person's energetic constitution. According to Thai medicine, everything, including our bodies, is composed of 4 types of energy: Earth (Din), Water (Nam), Fire (Fai) and Wind (Lom). Each person is born with a particular conjugation of these elements. Wherever there is an imbalance in one or some of these elements in us, illness appears. Thai massage as a therapy aims to balance the energy to achieve a state of health.

CHAPTER 2
WAI KRUU

Within the Thai massage field there is a ritual that the Thais perform just before the massage begins. It is called wai kruu. The wai kruu is an invocation, a mantra in honor of Dr. Shivago, considered the father of Thai medicine. This title comes from the fact that Shivago was Buddha's personal physician. Because Thailand is a Buddhist country, Dr. Shivago is considered a patron of all those who are engaged in the practice of any branch of medicine, including, of course, massage therapy. Some masseurs recite an abbreviated version of the mantra before each treatment. Below is a Romanesque transcription of the mantra in Pali, with its translation into English.

PRAYER TO INVITE **the spirit of the Father of Medicine Dr. Shivago**

OM NAMO SHIVAGO SIRASA A-HANG

KARUNIKO SPPASATANANG O-SATHA
TIPPAMANTANG PAPHASO SURIYAJANTANG
KOMARAPATO PAGASESI WANTAMI
BANTITO SUMETASO A-LOKA SUMANAHOMI
PIYO-TEWA MANUSANANG PIYO-PROMMA
NUMUTTAMO PIYO-NAKA SUPANNANANG
PININSRIYONG NAMAMIHANG NAMOPUTAYA
NAVON-NAVEAN NAVAE NAPAITANGVEAN
NAVEANMAHAKU A-HIMAMA PIYONGMAMA
NAMOPUTTAYA
NA-A NAVA OKA PAYATI INASANTI

TRANSLATION:

> We invite the spirit of our founder, Father Dr.
> Shivagokomarpaj, who will come to us
> through his holy life. Please give us the
> knowledge of nature.
> May this prayer reveal the true medicine of
> the universe.
> In the name of this prayer, we respect your
> help and pray that through our bodies
> you may bring wellness and health to our
> patients. The god of healing dwells above
> in the heavens while humanity remains
> below it.
> In the name of the Founder, may the heavens
> be reflected on Earth, so that this healing
> medicine may envelop the world.
> We pray for the one whom we touch, that he
> may be happy and free from all sickness.

We should not be surprised if we find other different

translations, since the average Thai does not speak Pali, as this language, which derives from Sanskrit, is used exclusively in religious ceremonies, in the same way that Latin was used in ancient Catholic mass. On the other hand, its importance does not lie in its exact translation, but in its purpose, which is the mental and spiritual preparation, both for receiving the teachings of the technique and for practicing the massage. Ultimately, what is sought is to direct the mind into the sacred in order to sacralize the therapeutic work and thus detach from the ego and become an instrument of higher forces. In my opinion, the mantra is ultimately a vehicle, an instrument, a form. I believe that sticking to traditional wai kruu makes sense for people with an inclination towards Buddhism, for the rest, it may be insipid or meaningless. For this reason I prefer to teach my students to create their own version of wai kruu. It doesn't have to be a long prayer, it doesn't even have to be a prayer. As long as it is something that connects the practitioner to his or her most spiritual and sacred part, it will be fine. You can visualize the image of a saint, a guru, or simply an image or sound that induces us to feel peace or selfless love. I believe that the wai kruu takes on its true purpose when we adapt it to our way of understanding and perceiving spirituality. So, if your heart is in Buddhism, the Pali mantra can fulfill its function, if you are a Christian the image of Christ or the Lord's Prayer, if you are a Hindu the image of Shiva or Krishna, or perhaps the Om symbol or sound. What is important in the end is the essence, so whatever the form, if you achieve a state of peace and connection with the sacred in you, you will be performing the wai kruu correctly.

CHAPTER 3
BEFORE STARTING THE PRACTICE

Before moving on to the more practical part of this book, we must review an important concept, that of general massage vs. therapeutic massage. Why is this important?

Because most schools confuse theory with practice, that is, they teach the practical part as if it were a rigid theory with no possibility of modification.

MANY TIMES I have been told: "Cesar, I went to this place and there I had to memorize the protocol, and if I skipped a maneuver or performed it at another part of it during the massage, they would lower my score." To which I always answer: "I will lower your score if you follow the protocol exactly as I taught it."

This is because the key to Thai massage as a treatment is in the personalization, in making a different and unique massage according to the client and the situation.

. . .

YOU HAVE to analyze the characteristics and needs of the client and know the maneuvers very well to be able to do a massage that fits what the person needs. General massage is useful as a relaxation treatment for people who are already well, but it loses a lot of potential with those who really need a massage. To get the most out of this style, one must begin to become familiar with the technique. This is where we find the real function of the general protocol. Thai massage is not a sequence of movements, massage is an art, and as such, it gives us the ability to create. The reason for the protocol is to function as an excuse to incorporate the technique. When you practice a certain protocol over and over again, you are habituating your body to a new way of moving, to a new way of relating to the client's body, to see what sensations it provokes. Hence the protocol is, in fact, extremely necessary. But only until you has understood the how, when, why and for whom of each technique. Once this has been achieved, it is necessary to disarticulate the protocol in multiple ways. That is to say, change the order of the manipulations, eliminate technique, add techniquess, etc.

FOR THIS REASON AT SHIVATHAI, the course is composed of 11 protocols and I instruct on how to combine them in the best way according to the type of client. There is also an element that I consider very important, and that is how the technique affects me according to the difference in physique and weight between the client and me as a therapist. This is for me the best way to do massage because if you only concentrate on the client, sooner or later you will find that the massage you do can help the client but it can also affect your health if you do not choose the right techniques. By keeping this element in mind, you can create a session that is good for the client and also helps you to continue in the profession for decades, without joint problems, tendonitis or back pain as many massage therapists suffer from. That said, I invite you to move on to the practical part, knowing that you will be practicing it as is, to gain skill and confidence. Although you are a beginner, it does not mean that you will not see results, you will see them, but keep in mind that at this stage the most important thing is to learn, gain mastery and get to feel comfortable with the movements. Let's get down to work.

PART II
PRACTICE

"When you touch a body, you touch the whole person, his intellect, his spirit, and his emotions.."

— JANE HARRINGTON

This is where we are going to get into doing massage. Although the protocol is simple, some techniques may not feel comfortable and/or you may feel clumsy. Don't worry, this is normal. It is important to remember that you are learning something new and allowing yourself to hesitate and move with difficulty. No one is born knowing, and even the most basic techniques may seem difficult at first. Don't be discouraged if this happens to you. Give your body time to get used to being on the ground. In Part III of the book you will find some tips for coping with some common problems that can arise with practice.

Let's get started.

CHAPTER 4
THERAPIST'S POSTURES

All right, now that we are going to start practicing the massage, let's first do a brief review of the basic postures of the therapist. Sometimes people contact me saying they have this or that physical problem and want to know if they can do Thai massages. An easy way to find out is this: if you can get in the following postures, you can do a massage. If you find one or more of these postures difficult, it does not mean that you are not suitable for massage, you will simply have to gradually get your body used to the posture until you feel comfortable in it. This is achieved through time, dedication and practice. In my years as a trainer I have seen many cases of people having difficulty with posture or displacement, but with tenacity and patience they manage to overcome the difficulty and do the massage without problems. So if you feel that any posture causes you discomfort or pain, do not be discouraged, the body is malleable and will adapt according to what you need to do with it if you work hard enough.

Now, let's go to the positions:

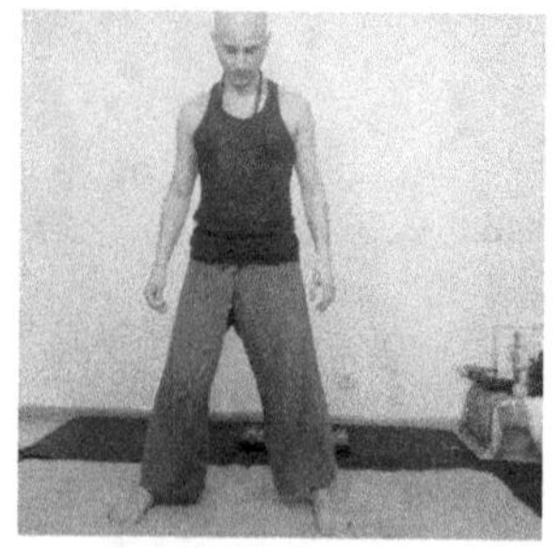

STANDING POSTURE: This may seem simple, but keep in mind that it is a massage posture, so if you have one or both feet on top of the client, you will need some concentration and practice to maintain balance and know how to transmit the proper weight to each person.

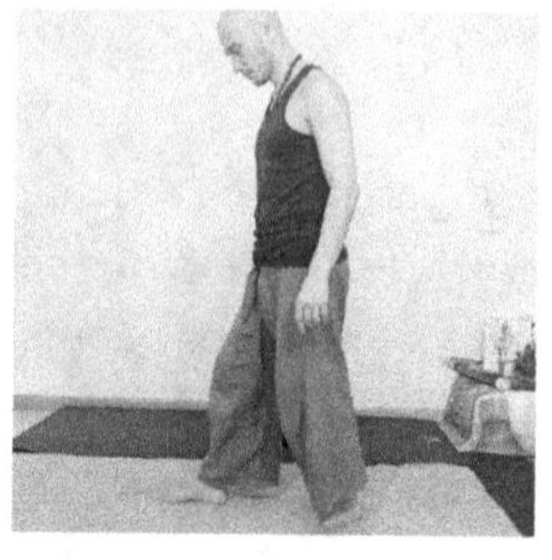

TAICHI: Same observation as in the previous posture. You have to know how to graduate the pressure according to the person and the part of the body you are touching. To know how to distribute your weight properly you must know how to work with your axis and master your balance and coordination. Your feet can become a great tool because you can massage people with big, heavy bodies without getting tired. If you are inexperienced and lack balance, a good way to work with this posture is to rest one or both hands on a chair, a bar or side bars, or on the ceiling, or on a wall or piece of furniture.

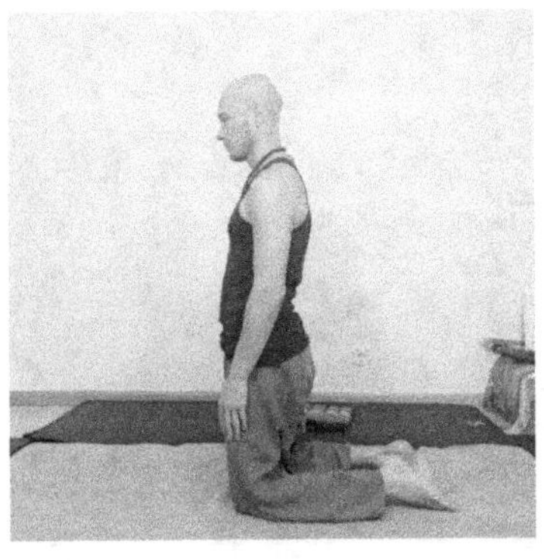

Kneeling: this position can be used to exert a strong pressure wherever you decide to lean (I like to use it to work on the legs of very large people). It will also help you perform some passive stretching.

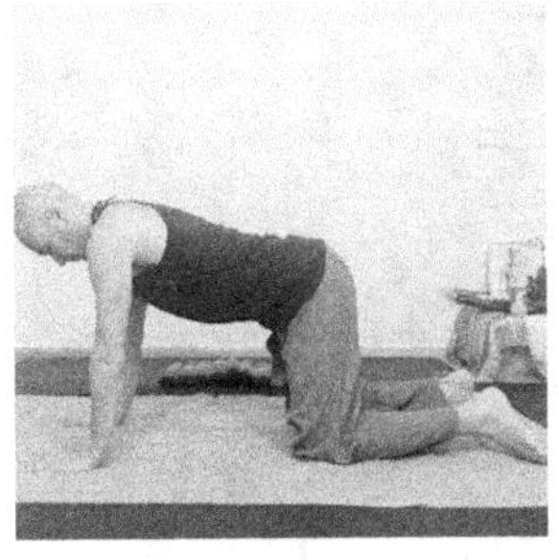

THE CAT: this is an interesting posture because it can serve as a support while using your hands, or as a working tool, i.e., you can reverse the function and place your hands on the floor while resting your knees on some part of the body to exert compression. You can also do compression using the knees and hands at the same time (for example, placing the knees behind the buttocks while doing palm presses on the back).

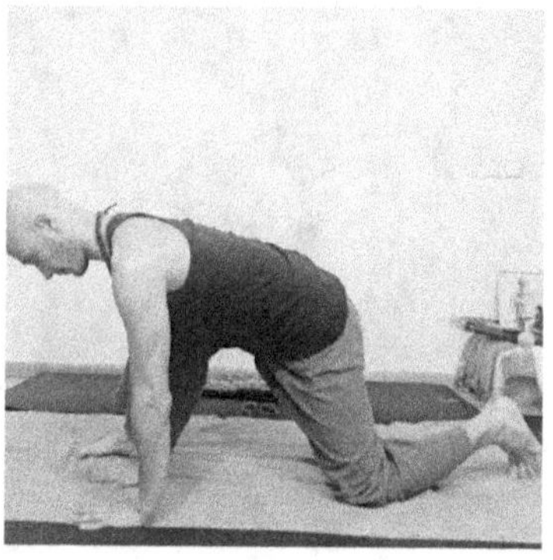

WARRIOR POSE: This is one of the most common postures in this style. We will use it to do palm and digital walks, pressures of all kinds, as well as to move around the client.

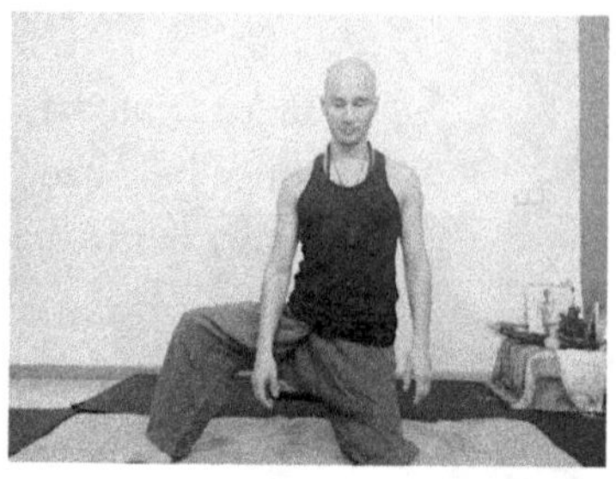

OPEN WARRIOR: We will use this posture to do compressions and as an aid to perform certain manipulations of the recipient's body. Very useful, for example, to do palmar and/or digital walks on the recipient's back, with the foot on one side of the body and the knee on the other while doing alternating or simultaneous compressions along the back.

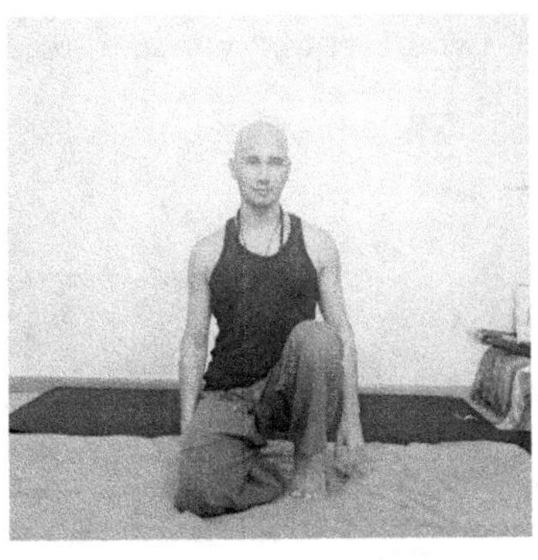

Archer pose: used to perform various passive stretches.

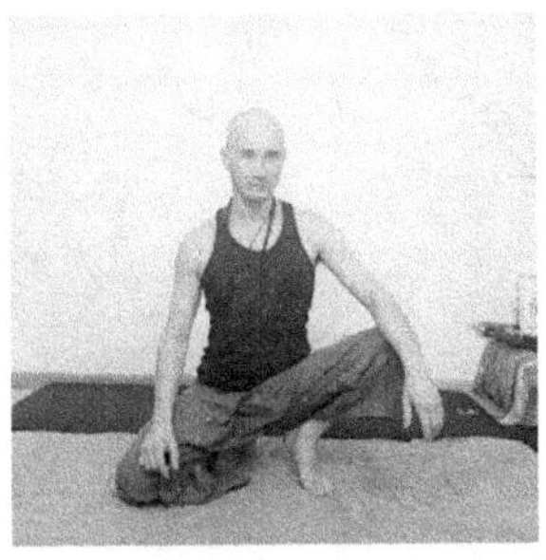

OPEN ARCHER : this is a variant of the previous one, and is used for the same purposes. The best way to know which is the most optimal is simply to try one or the other posture and see which one is more comfortable for the maneuver we wish to perform. Here again, the size difference between the person receiving and the therapist comes into play.

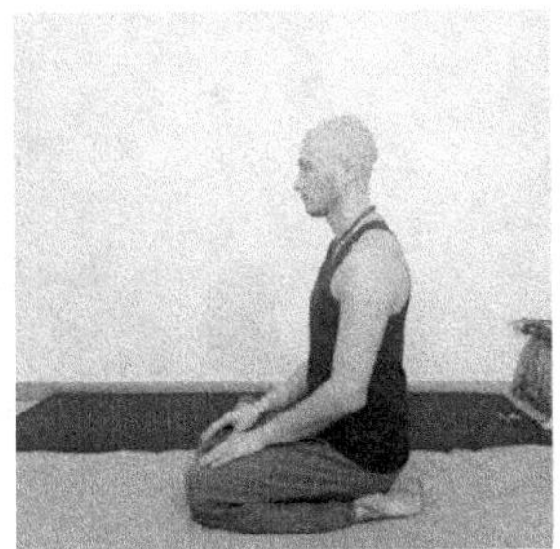

DIAMOND POSE: used as a starting position at the beginning of the massage, but also as a position to perform other techniques. The interesting thing about this position is that it is quite comfortable when you get used to it, and you feel that you can "rest" while you are doing the massage.

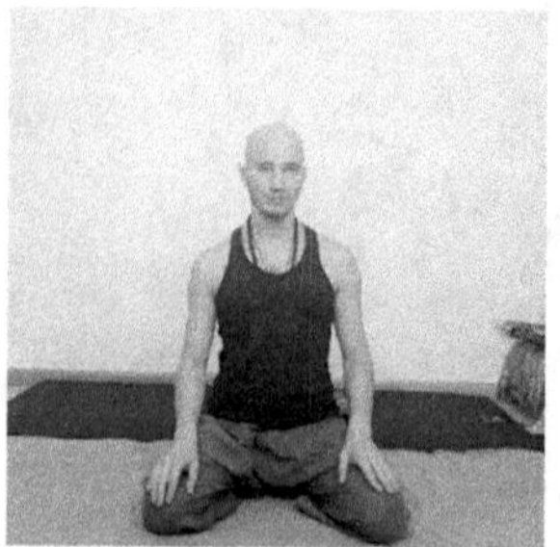

OPEN DIAMOND: it is a variant of the previous one and is used for the same purpose.

CHAPTER 5
THE MINIMUM VIABLE
MASSAGE

In my third or fourth year as a Thai masseur, I started to feel very comfortable with this style. As a result, I wanted to learn more and better techniques. My sessions started to become more complex in terms of technique, that is, I included a lot of movements throughout the massage session. I never counted them, but I knew that while the massage lasted, I would take my client from one posture to another and I would perform an endless number of different techniques with the objective of making my treatments more and more efficient. Then the trips came, the possibilities for learning new styles, meeting different masters, and learning even more.

A few years after that, I began to feel that perhaps there was no need for so many movements in the session. Not even a variety of techniques. Then I began to elaborate a minimalist massage, a massage that, with a few maneuvers, could have the same effect as applying Pareto's law[1].

It all started when I began working with another therapist who was a friend. She was a Thai masseuse and yoga teacher, and she was the most flexible person I had ever met. Having a similar professional profile to mine, having studied with several of my own teachers, I wanted to make every session amazing for her, and I wanted to make her feel the power of an advanced Thai massage session.

We worked together for a whole year until she went on a trip. A year later she came back and contacted me to continue with the project. This time I decided to put the experiment into practice, even though her body was still extremely flexible and strong, and knowing how well she had responded the whole year I worked with her, I decided to change my strategy. I would do a minimalist, simplified session, a minimum viable massage, as I would later call it. Something in me had changed, I felt a certain maturity professionally speaking, which allowed me to achieve a lot with very little. And so it was, after that session my friend told me how much she liked it, and that she felt a very deep effect on her, both physically and emotionally.

What I did was basically a protocol with the simplest techniques, very calmly and repeating them over and over again. No rush, no need to demonstrate anything, no advanced postures or complicated sequences. Just compressions, acupressure, mobilization, some stretching, nothing else. And it worked so well that from then on, each session would be more or less similar: 3 or 4 techniques, 1 or 2 stretches, no more than that. A very simple session, but with a deep and healing effect.

Although today I still enjoy doing sessions with many movements, complex structures and advanced techniques, I still perform the minimum viable massage that is for me the ultimate way to go to the next level. When you set out to fix a client's problem with a few movements, you have to know the technique, your body, the client, and the size difference between the two well enough to achieve an efficient, quality massage session.

The minimum viable massage is effective and fulfills its purpose when the therapist has gone through a process of learning and mastering the technique, when one is able to refine his/her "clinical eye" and know which techniques will be best for the client.

The protocol you will see below is a minimum viable massage for you, a massage with just the right techniques to relieve the tension and pain of most people who suffer from typical stress and muscle tension caused by a sedentary life-style. The purpose of this protocol is to take those first important steps when you want to acquire a new skill, that you go from inaction to action through a sequence of movements that are easy to learn and that in turn have a great impact on the health of the people you touch.

If you came up to this book because you wanted to learn, that's great, once you do that I invite you to unlearn what you have learned. I mean, once you feel comfortable with the technique and you know the protocol by heart, try changing the order of the sequences, changing the order of the movements, remove techniques, add techniques, in short, destroy the protocol and create something new. Then pay attention to the person you are going to work on, and ask yourself: do I really need to do this stretching? Do I need to spend a lot of time on this person's feet or legs? Is an abdominal massage indispensable in this case considering the time I have and the priority of the receiver? By putting these ideas into practice in your massage session, you will be ready for the next step, but for now, let's concentrate on this one -- the protocol.

1. Principle elaborated by the Italian economist Vilfredo Pareto in which he describes that 80% of the results come from 20% of the efforts. This rule is also known as the 80/20 principle.

CHAPTER 6
PREPARATION

You may not need this chapter; you may be already fit and flexible. In this case let's just go directly to the next chapter where we will start with the protocol.

If, on the other hand, you consider yourself a person with no elasticity and you have never done body work on the floor, I advise you to stay to see some very simple exercises that will make your life easier when doing the massage.

WHEN I STARTED Thai massage I was 25 years old, and I had been training martial arts for 12 years, you could say that my body was well trained, I had no major difficulty getting used to the movements necessary for this work, and I definitely did not lack flexibility.

You don't need to have the flexibility of a dancer or martial artist. Whatever age you are and whatever state you are in, you can do Thai massage sessions if you have the desire to learn, the time to devote to practice, and someone to model for you. That's all. You have to understand that when you start a new activity, the body will offer some resistance, precisely because it is doing something it is unfamiliar with. Therefore, it is to be expected that you may not feel comfortable with certain postures or movements. The body is more malleable than you think, and if you practice and give it enough time, your body will adjust to the new activity. Remember this:

"It is difficult until it is no longer so."

All right, now I will show you a series of basic exercises to get your body used to the kind of movement you'll do and make everything easier for you.

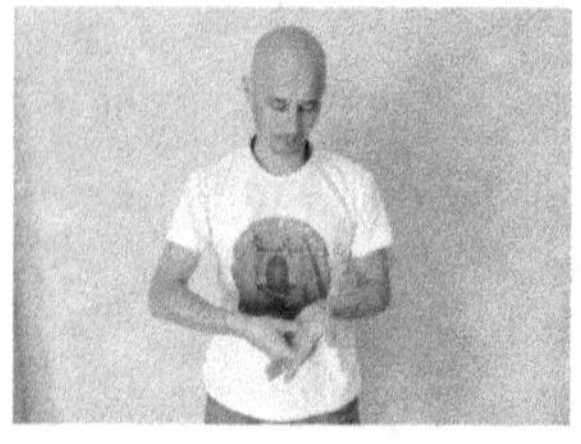

1-**CIRCULAR MASSAGE at the center of the palm.** We are going to interlace the fingers and create circular friction with the thumb. This is very important because we will work with palm pressure a lot during the massage, this massage technique will help us increase blood flow in the area and improve our sensitivity.

2-**FINGER STRETCH:** Stretch the arm forward, palm facing forward and fingers down. With our other hand, we take the fingertips and pull them towards us. This is useful for making the wrist and fingers more flexible and stretching the muscles of the forearm. At first it may be uncomfortable,

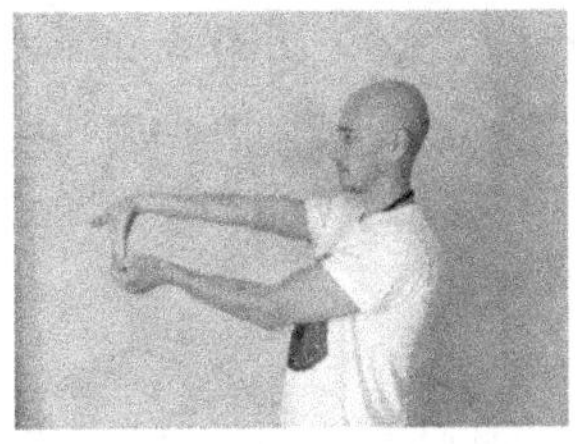

but it will help us get our hands used to the contact position in the pressure.

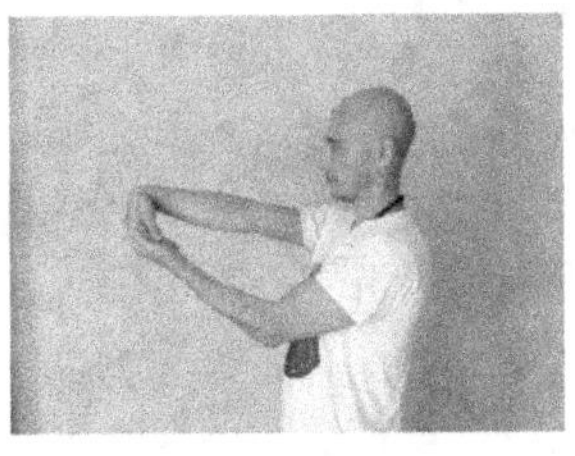

3-**WRIST FLEXION:** Same position as above, but this time with the palm facing up. We take the back of the hand and pull in our direction until we feel that it is enough. It is important that we stretch slowly and smoothly.

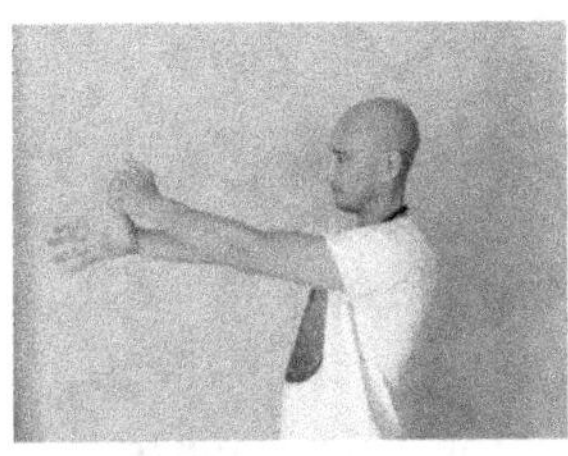

4-**THUMB FLEXION.** Arm and fingers forward, we take the thumb and pull backwards. With this we improve our mobility and relax the finger that we use the most in the massage session.

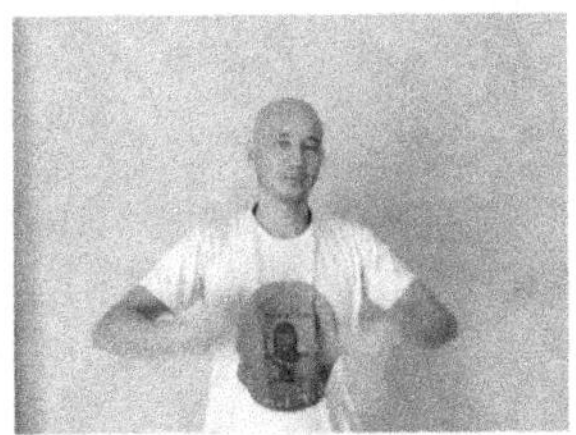

5-**WE LOOSEN our hands and move our arms around.** We do this with an up and down movement, with relaxed wrists and fingers, as if we were splashing water. This helps release tension in the hands and the muscles of our fingers. Although we are using a pre-massage routine, you can do this exercise after the session if you feel overloaded, you will notice the difference and your hands will thank you.

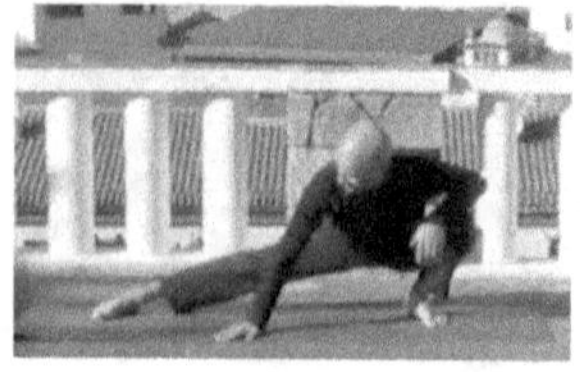

6-**Dragon stretch**: Now we are going to work a little on leg flexibility. We separate our feet to double shoulder width and bend one leg while keeping the soles of our feet on the floor. If you notice any of your feet lifting, lift your hips back up and keep the soles of your feet flat on the floor. You can place your hands on the floor. Bounce very softly and slowly, feeling your body weight lower and stretching it out a bit. Perform 5-10 bounces and then repeat on the other side.

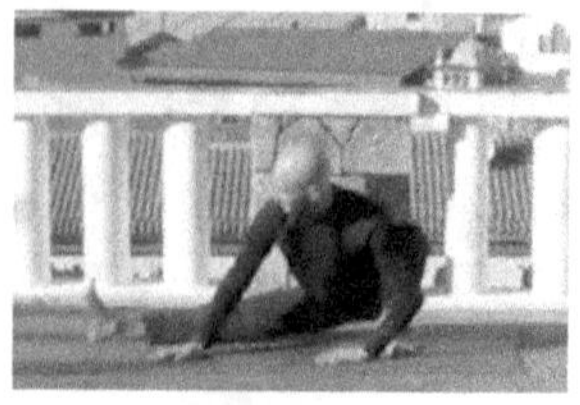

7-**Dragon stretch II**: We do the same as in the previous exercise, but this time the foot of the stretched leg rests on the heel instead of the sole. The toe of the foot is pointing in an upward direction. The rule of thumb for knowing if you are stretching well is very simple: if you feel a bearable pain, it is fine, if it does not hurt at all, it means that you are not going down far enough, or you have to perform a more advanced stretch. If it hurts too much, you should make it softer.

8-**Front stretch**: We move one foot forward and the other one backwards, supporting the metatarsus on the floor. We lower the body with a soft, slow bounce, as in the

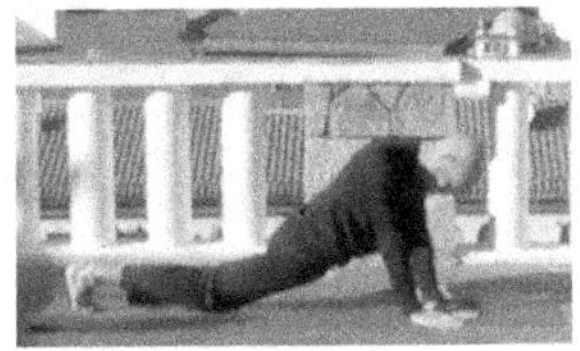

previous exercise. Repeat on the other side.

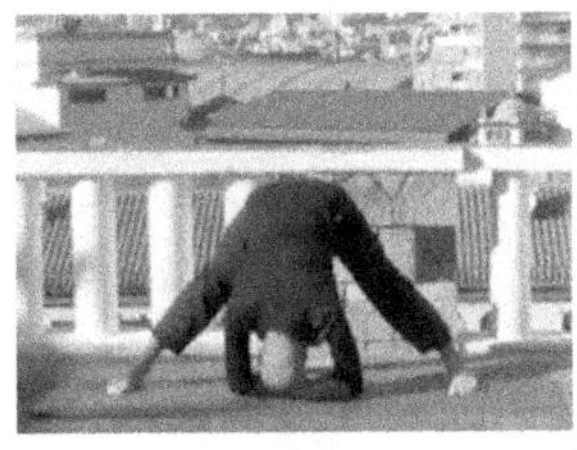

9-HANGING THE TRUNK: We open the legs at double shoulder width, lower the trunk down slowly, interlace the arms above the head and hold the position for a few seconds. The arms can be intertwined or just hanged. The back, neck and head also hang. Just feel the back stretching, take 5 to 10 deep breaths and then slowly come back to the original position until you are back up.

THESE MOVEMENTS SERVE as preparation and warm-ups. You can perform them every day at first, and then only once in a while if you have any other exercises or stretching routines or do yoga.

CHAPTER 7
SEQUENCE A: PRONE POSITION

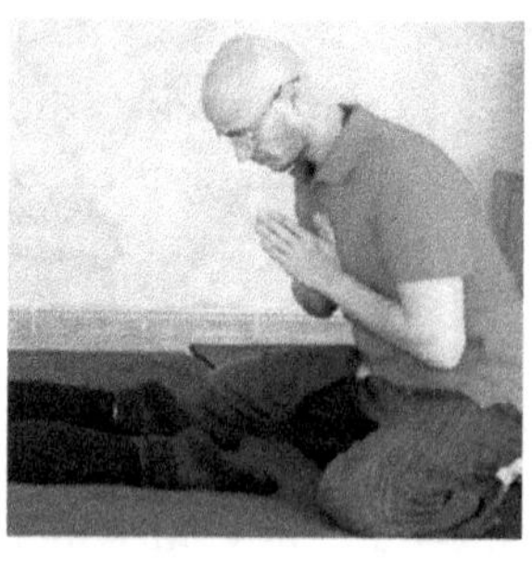

1-Wai kruu

Let's start with this ritual called wai kruu. Remember that in Thailand it is performed by reciting a mantra in Pali that we saw in another chapter, but it is sacred to you to put your hands together at the level of your heart and bow.

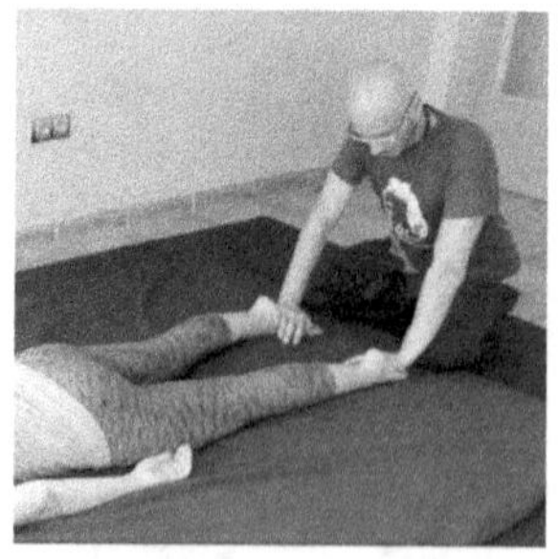

2-PALM PRESSURE **on feet**

While we rest the palms of our hands on the person's feet, it is important to keep our arms straight because they will allow us to transmit our weight. We maintain contact for a few seconds, and then we begin to rock our bodies gently to the sides, to load weight on the heels of our hands alternately, in different parts of the soles of the feet of the client. This helps to start with relaxation, and also gives us an idea of the client's level of flexibility. If the heels yield easily to the floor, the client will almost certainly have good flexibility, and if there is a lot of resistance, he or she will probably suffer from some stiffness. In this case, it would be advisable to place a roller on the bottom of both ankles.

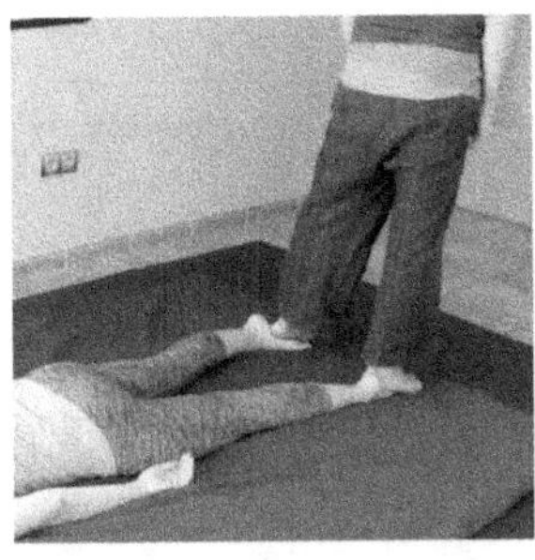

3-FOOT PRESSURE on the feet

We stand up and place our heels in the center of the client's soles, swinging our weight from one foot to the other. This part of the body can usually hold a lot of pressure easily, but I advise you to ask the person how he/ she feels about the pressure. This technique helps relieve stress. It is also a technique to have in mind because the wear and tear on the therapist is virtually zero. So if you have a very large client or you have a lot of appointments in a day, or you are just not very energetic one day, it is a good strategy to use this technique to manage your energy. It can also be done on the palms of the hands and other parts of the body.

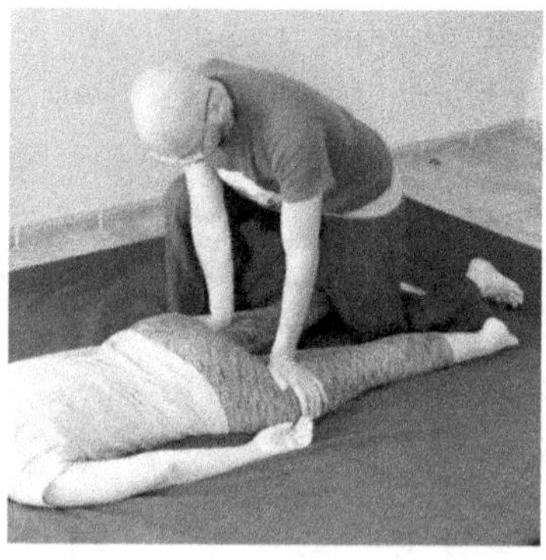

4-PALMAR WALKING **on legs**

Here we are going to do an alternating palmar pressure up and down the legs, as if we were walking. This helps to improve circulation and relieve the leg pain and stiffness. It is a basic but very effective technique for people who are on their feet all day, athletes and people with circulation issues.

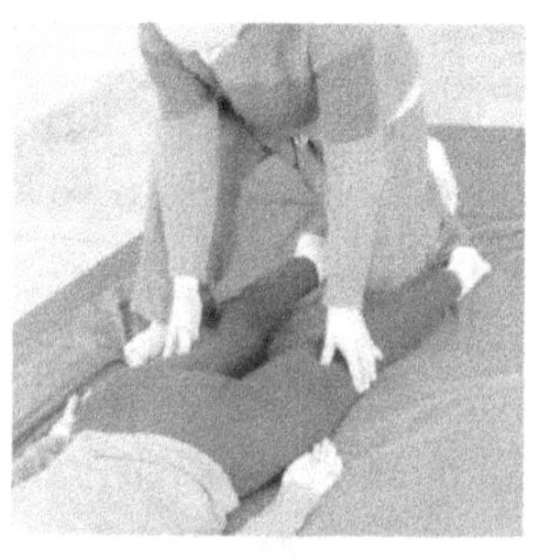

5-THUMB **and palm walk on legs**

Now let's do another walk back and forth, this time with the thumb over the midline of the leg, from the Achilles tendon to the ischium, between 6 and 8 points along the leg, avoiding the popliteal fossa (the area behind the knee). This technique promotes circulation and helps to eliminate adhesion. When you reach the feet again, repeat the palmar walk. It is important to understand that the pressure is on the pad of the thumb, not the tip. It is also important to pay attention to the rhythm. Some people tend to change the cadence of the movement when going from Palm to digital presses or vice versa. Maintaining a steady rhythm is vital to help the client relax and enjoy even more.

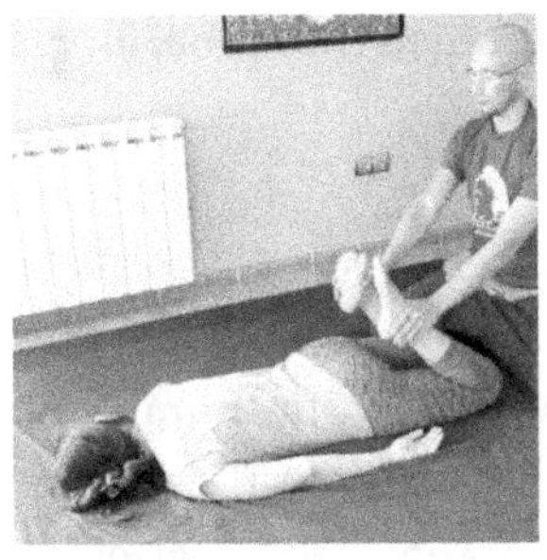

6-HEELS to gluteus

We take the feet and bring the heels down to the buttocks, first with parallel feet, and then with crossed feet. Then we stretch the legs again. With this movement you can assess the receiver's level of flexibility and stretch the quads. This is important because it allows you to build the protocol as you get more information from the client. So, if the client is heavier than you and this maneuver offers a lot of resistance, you will have to take this into account to evaluate what to do next, so that it is not too heavy for you and not too painful for the client.

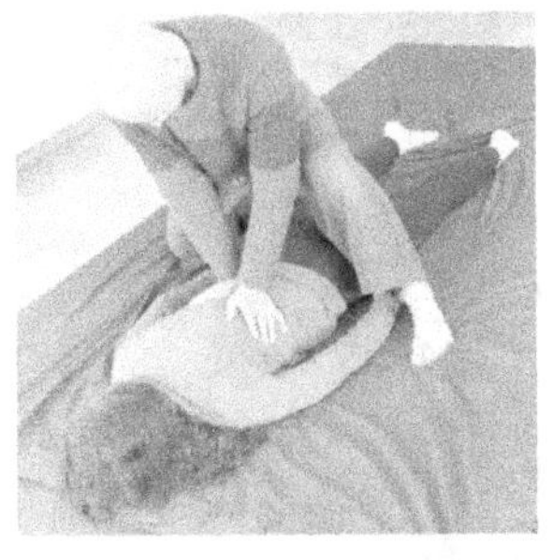

7-PALM WALK on the back

We go up with Palmar walking on the legs, and when we reach the gluteal line, we change position and continue with the Palmar walk on the back. In other words, we move from warrior to open warrior, with one knee on one side and one foot on the other. I recommend resting the hands on the legs, behind the buttocks, or on the sacrum, which are areas where the body can unload weight without problems and will make the change in posture more fluid.

With this technique we will see how the muscles and the spine are doing, and at the same time we can begin to relieve tension.The pressure goes from the lumbar to the scapular area. There are between 3 and 4 points of contact. Make sure that the heels of the hands are very close to the spine, along the paravertebral muscles.

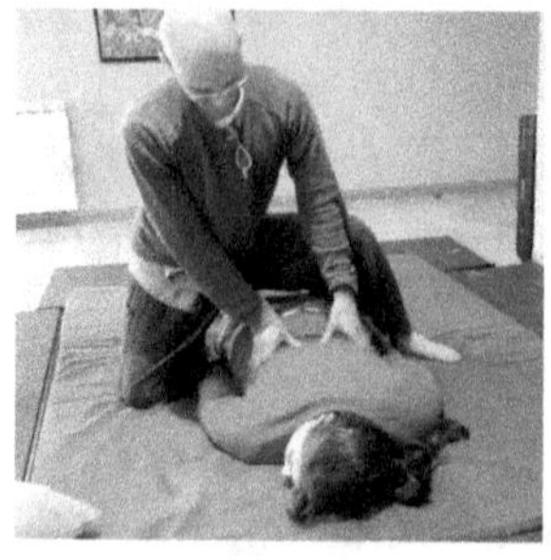

8-Thumb-walk on lines 1 and 2

We make an alternating pressure (walk) with thumbs on line 1, which is right next to the spine, between the vertebral processes and the paravertebral muscle, and you will notice a space, a kind of channel, between the vertebral processes and the paravertebral muscle. We will be doing 6 to 8 points of pressure from the lumbar to scapular area. Line 2 is right next to line 1, on the paravertebral muscle. The most common mistake I see is that people move too far away from line 2, so I recommend palpating the spine as a guide.

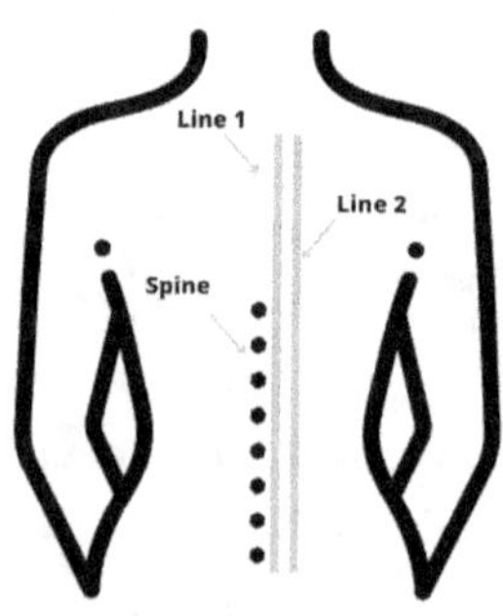

BACK LINES: Line 1, in the groove between the spine and the paravertebral muscle, on each side of the spine. Line 2, right on the paravertebral muscle.

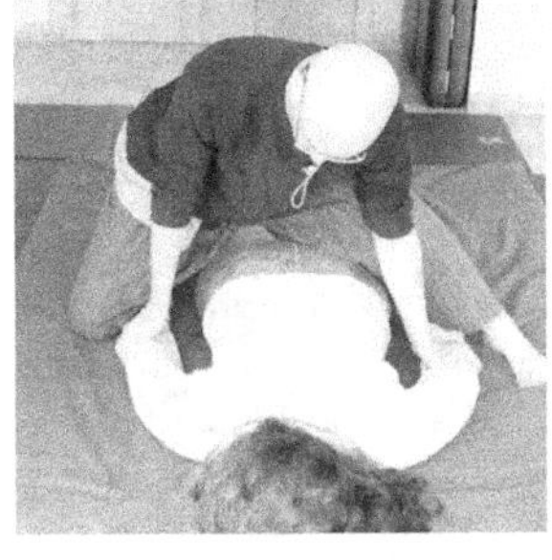

several more times.[1]

9-PALMAR WALKING on back and arms

We repeat the Palmar walk back and forth, then we go up again, this time down the arms to the hands. If we notice tension in the arms and forearms, we can repeat this walk

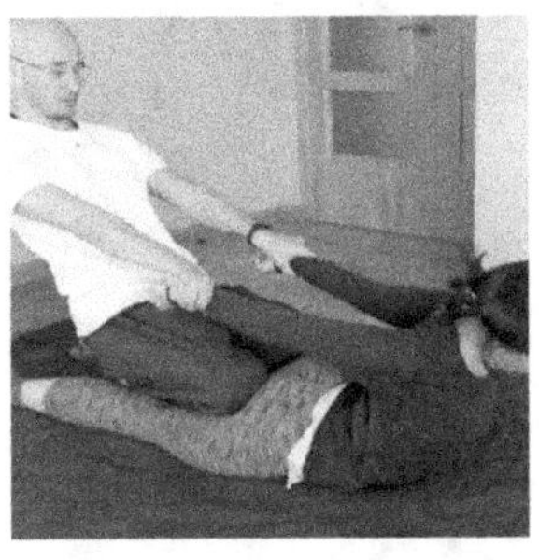

10-Cobra pose.

This is one of those classic Thai massage stretches. We take the client's wrists, ask the receiver to inhale, and tell him to exhale, and then pull our bodies backwards. This way we restore mobility to the back. If you are a yoga practitioner, you will notice that when you so this posture in a yoga class, you are told to inhale while going backwards, but this time you are asking the client to exhale. The objective of the technique is to restore mobility to the spine, which is easier when you exhale. It is not recommended in cases of hernias in the lumbar area.

11-RETURN TO FEET and ask the client to turn supine.

We go down with Palmar walking down the legs to the

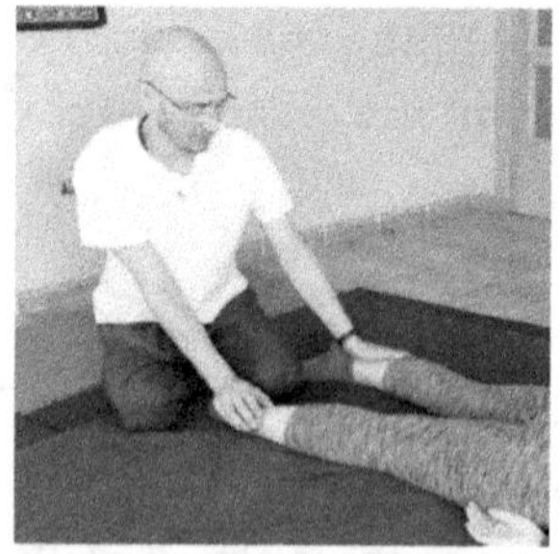

feet, and we ask the person to turn on his or her back. I recommend that you try to maintain a constant rhythm, this will improve the perception of the massage.

---

1. I say "we can" because everything will depend on our criteria. If you feel tension in the client's arms but you have little time, what you should do is dedicate yourself to work on what is most important for the receiver, that which is a priority.

CHAPTER 8
SEQUENCE B: SUPINE POSITION

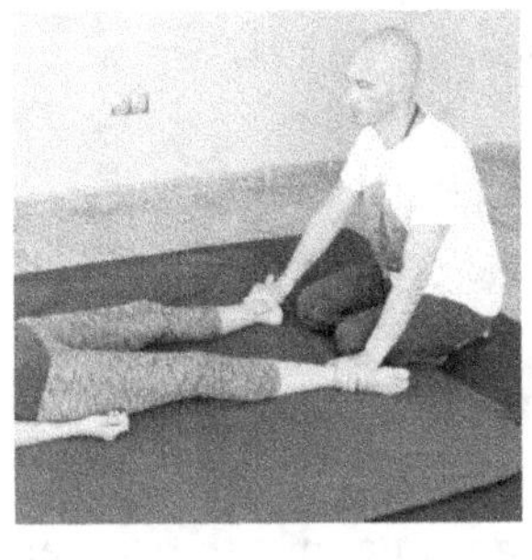

1-Alternate pressure on feet

With straight arms, swing your body slightly to shift the weight from one hand to the other. Watch the resistance of the client and don't force too much. The heels of the hands can be along the arch over the heels, and in the middle of the line if the client has flexibility.

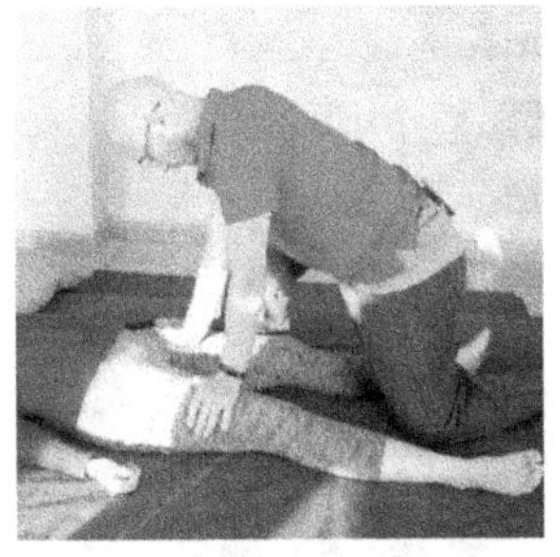

2-PALM WALK on legs

We go with alternating palmar pressure up the legs to the groin area back and forth. With this technique we improve circulation and we can observe the state of the muscle tissue as well as the pain tolerance level of the recipient. Recommendation: during this technique as in the others, you should pay attention to what you perceive while touching, look at the facial expression of the client, and in case you have any doubts, ask the client how they feel. This will help modulate the degree of pressure you apply.

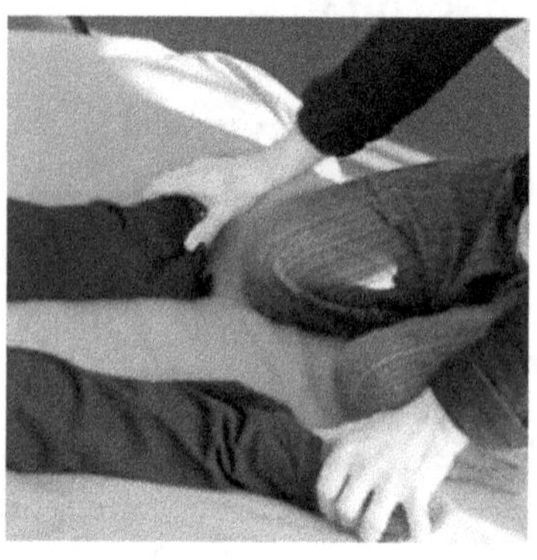

3-Thumb pressure on 2 lines of the foot

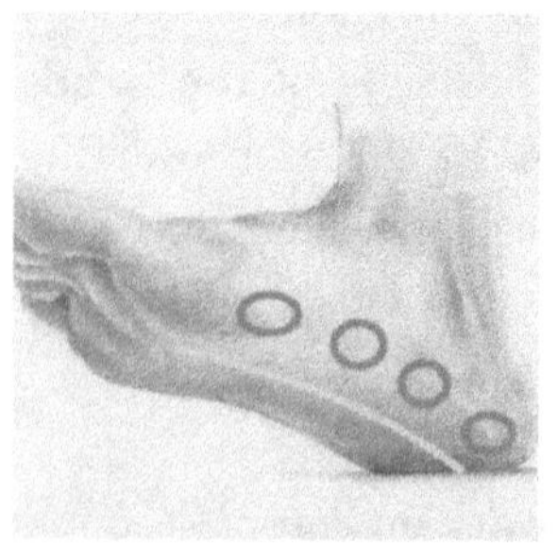

We walk with our thumbs on the arch line and the center line of the sole of the foot, and four points from the heel to just before the metatarsal. In particular, the arch line is very important because it is the reflex zone of the spine. This way, we are stimulating the back without touching it.

4-Circular knee movement

We take the foot, bend the leg and make circular movements to one side and the other to mobilize the knee. We

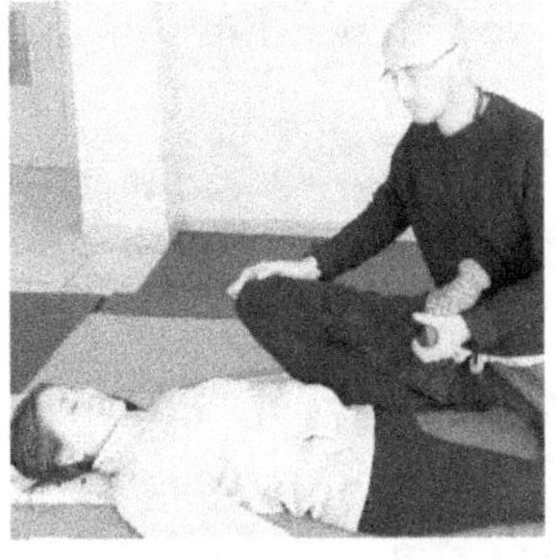

perform this movement 2 or 3 times per side for people with circulation problems and for sedentary people. For people with joint problems it is recommended to do it between 9 and 27 times.

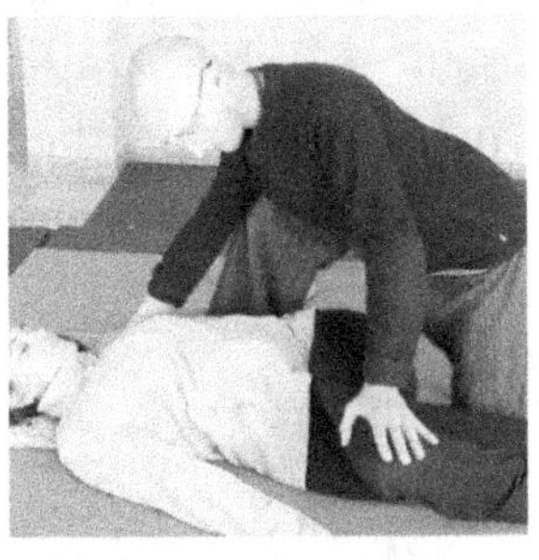

5-TORSION

We place the client's foot on the outside of the body, next to the opposite knee. With one hand on the shoulder and the other on the knee of the client, we press down to make a back twist. In this manner we restore mobility and intervertebral space to the client. For people with herniated discs in the lumbar area, you should avoid this technique or do it very carefully, gently and gradually.

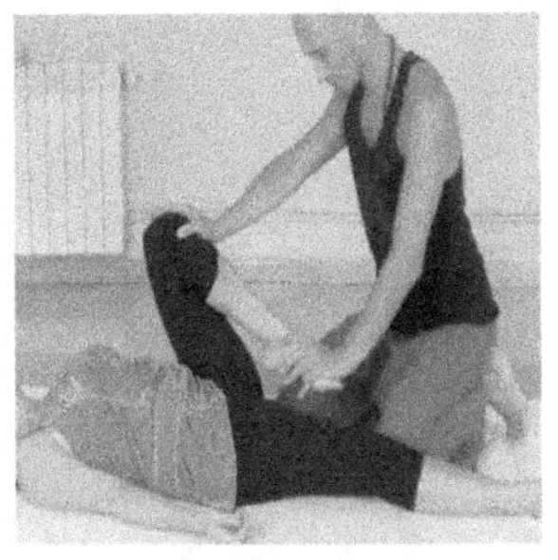

6-KNEE TO CHEST

We bring the knee of the client towards the chest, applying pressure on the instep, and bringing the heel towards the buttock at the same time. Be sure to keep your arms straight and swing your weight forward, this way you won't need to use force. You can be in a diamond, open diamond, kneeling or warrior position, whichever is more comfortable for you depending on the size of the receiver.

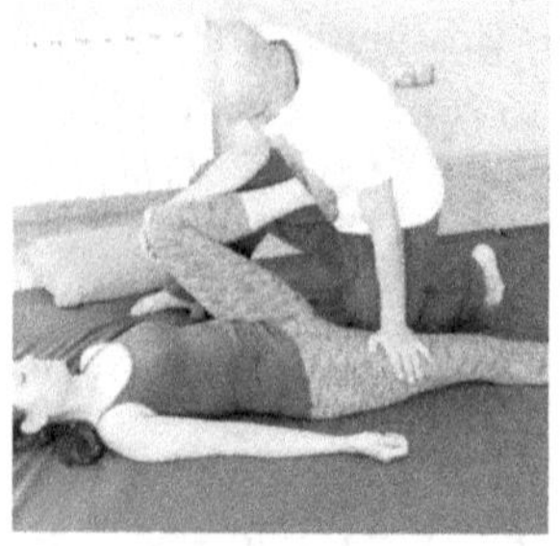

7-Da ku khaa

We place the client's foot on our hip, with one hand on the client's knee and the other on the straight leg. We rock our bodies back and forth, looking for resistance while also applying pressure on the other leg with the palm back and forth.

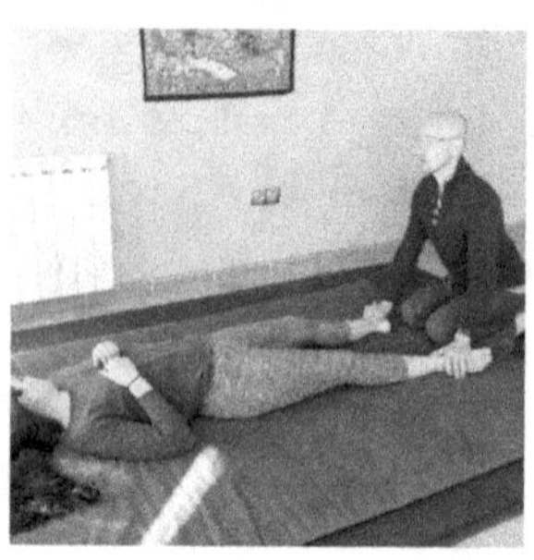

8-Return to feet.

Place the leg on the floor and repeat points 4 to 7 with the other leg. I recommend leaving the posture holding the leg from the heel and the popliteal hollow, that way we avoid the knee making an unpleasant bounce when we go backwards.

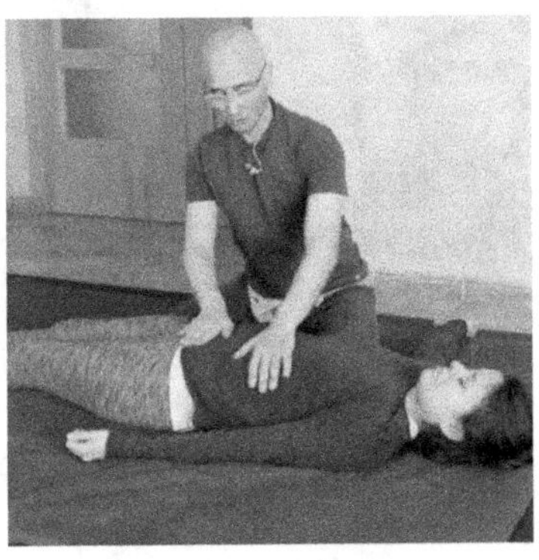

9-ABDOMEN: **friction**

From the feet, we go up with a palmar walk along the legs; when we reach the inguinal area, we place ourselves at the client's side in front of the abdominal area. We perform circular palmar friction in a clockwise direction. This helps to promote peristalsis.[1]

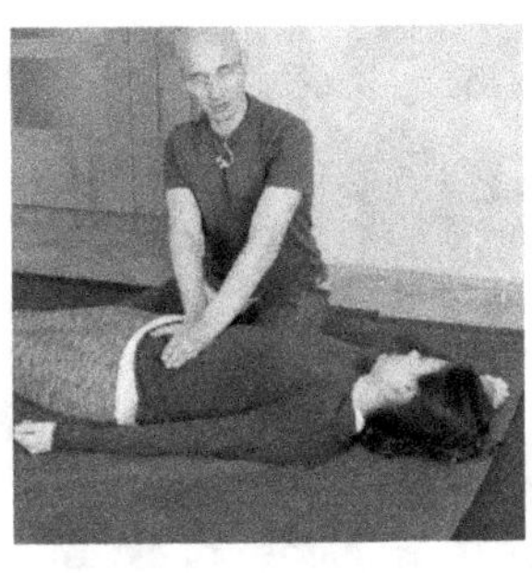

10-ABDOMEN: **the wave.**

We place one hand in front of the other on the navel line, the heel of the hand on one side, and the fingertips of our other hand on the other side of the abdomen. We perform a push-pull motion (slowly), like a wave, to mobilize tissue. This helps to stimulate the client's internal organs.

11-Abdomen: direct pressure

Put your hands together, the heel of the hand above the navel and apply direct pressure. We count 10 pulses and gradually release. We finish with circular friction again. This pressure must be deep, which

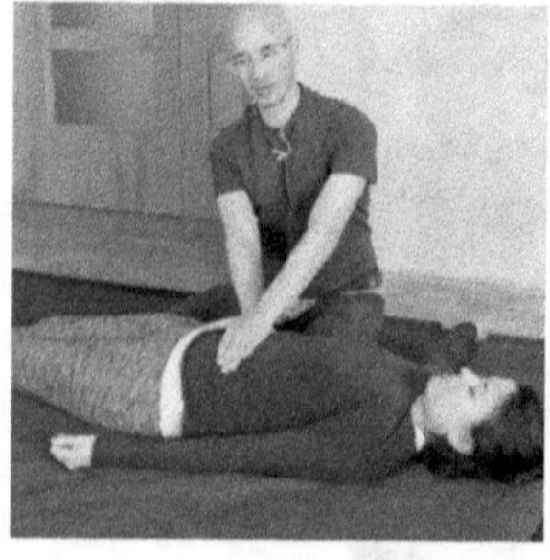

will almost certainly cause discomfort. I recommend watching the client's facial expression or asking him directly if he is okay and if he can hold it well. If the client feels the pressure is too much, loosen it a little to a level that is bearable for him.

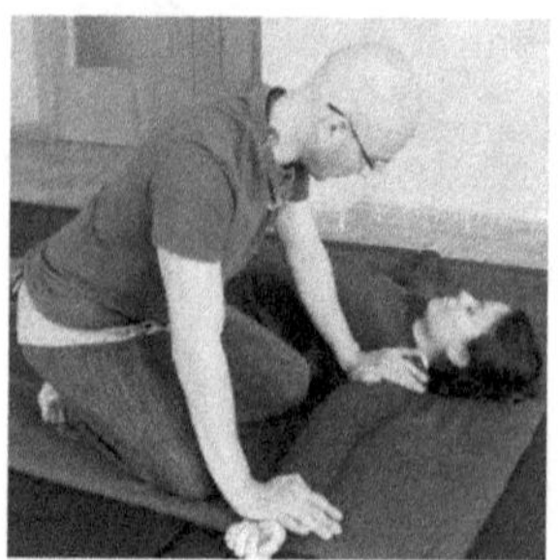

12-ARM STRETCHING.

We change position, with the client's arm open, we make a downward and slightly outward pressure, from the wrist to the armpit.

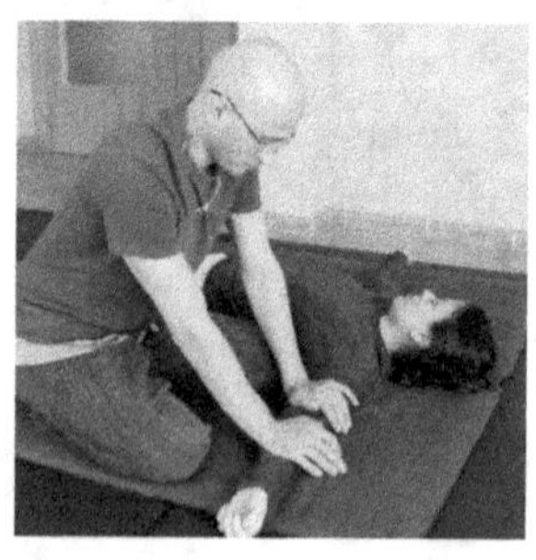

13-PALM PRESSURE.

We perform a palmar walk along the whole arm, from the inside to the outside or from the outside to the inside, back and forth. Two to three points of contact on each part of the arm (arm and forearm).

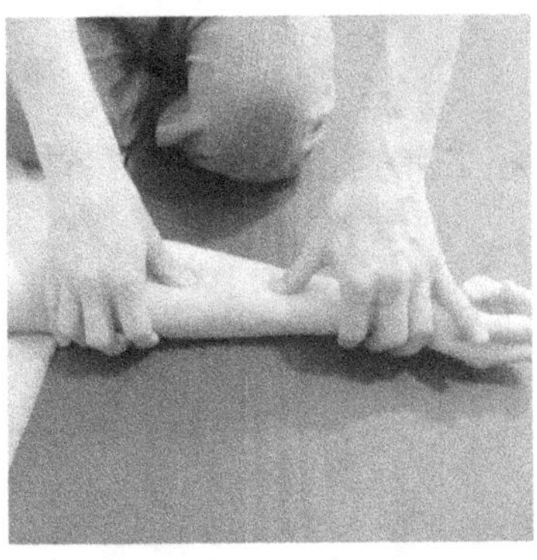

14-Thumb and palm walk.

We do another walk, this time with a thumb over the center line on the forearm and under the biceps on the arm, with three points of contact on each part of the arm. Back and forth, repeat the Palmar walk. Remember that the precise location of the points is not important, what is important to follow the line.

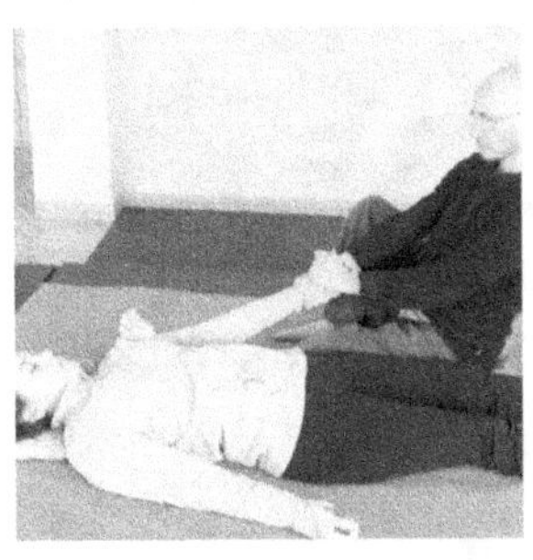

15-ARM STRETCHING 2.

We close the client's arm, grasp her hand and wrist with both hands, place our foot in her armpits and gently stretch once or twice. Try to place your foot slightly tilted instead of straight on the armpit.

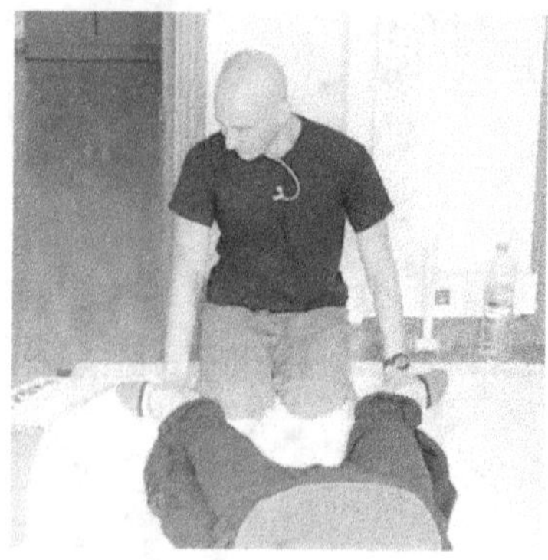

16-Change sides.

We work the other side of the body and repeat this from point 12 to 15. Then, with Palmar walking back to his feet. We spend a few moments doing alternating palmar pressure on the feet. This helps us evaluate what we have done so far and decide what to do next.

---

1. It is the bowel movement that carries fecal matter into the rectum and from there out of the body.

CHAPTER 9
SEQUENCE C: LATERAL AND SEATED

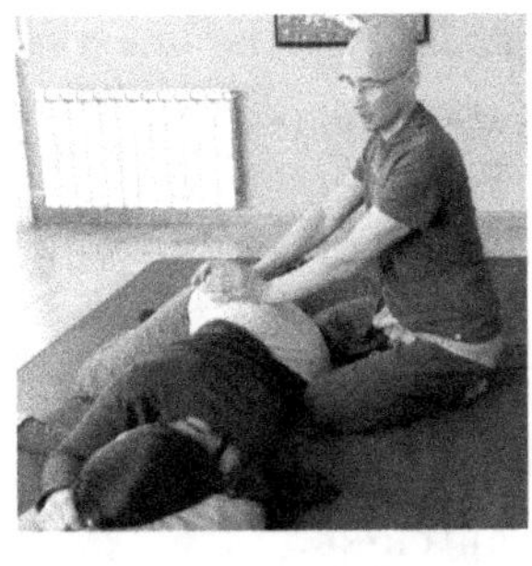

1-Presión palmar en glúteo, sacro y espalda

We ask the receiver to move to a lateral position. We go up the legs with a palmar walk and when we reach the hip, we move behind the client's back. Once there, we do alternating palmar pressure on the buttock, sacrum and back, always back and forth.

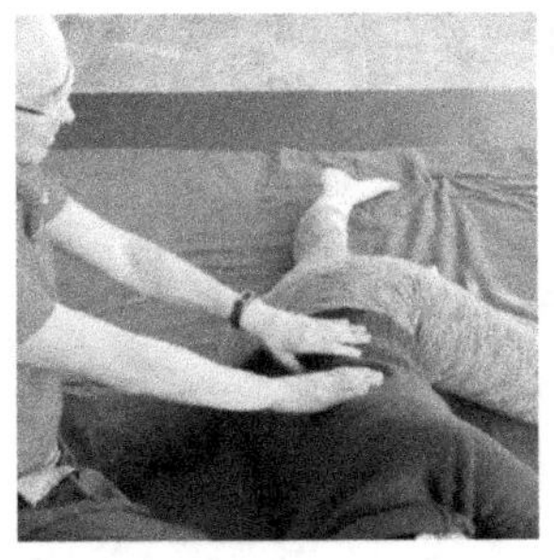

2-THUMB WALK ON LINE 1.

After the palmar walk we do a thumb walk on line 1 on the upper side of the back, above the vertebral process, before the paravertebral muscle, from the lumbar area to the middle of the scapular area, and we work between 6 and 8 points. Remember that this area has a groove that runs parallel to the spine. Your arms should be stretched and your body slightly inclined forward to enable you to use more of your bodyweight. You can work on more points, but you have to evaluate if it is worth it considering the time you have and the priority criteria you have chosen for the client.

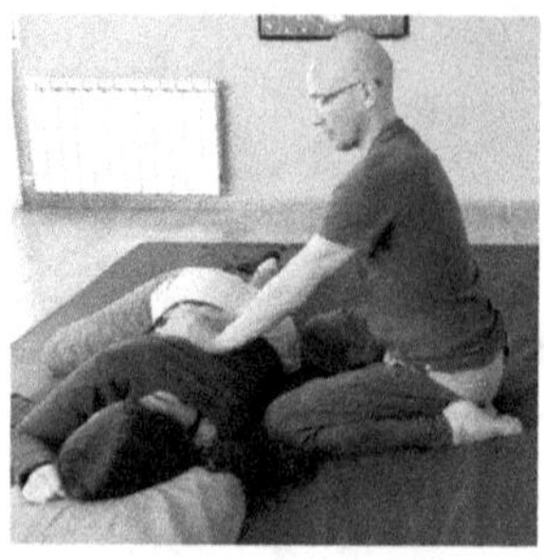

3-Thumb walk in line 2 + palmar walk.

We perform a thumb walk along the line 2 back and forth. Remember, line 2 is right next to line 1, right on the paravertebral muscle. We then repeat the palmar walk to soften the perception left by the thumb.

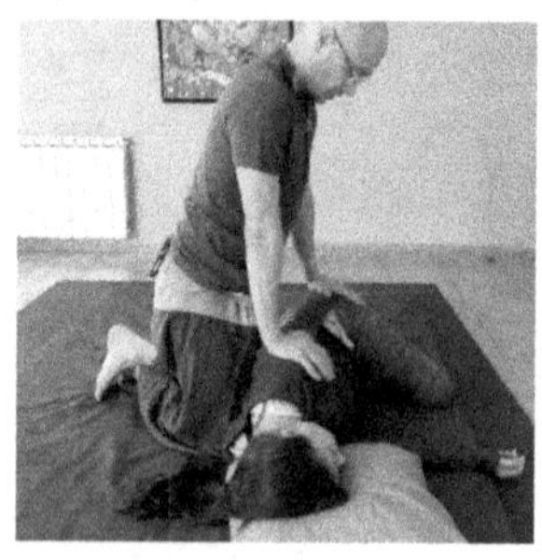

4-Arm stretching.

We place the arm over the client's body and apply pressure from wrist to shoulder. The pressure is inward and slightly outward.

5-Palm walk.

We perform a palm walk, from shoulder and wrist to the center back and forth.

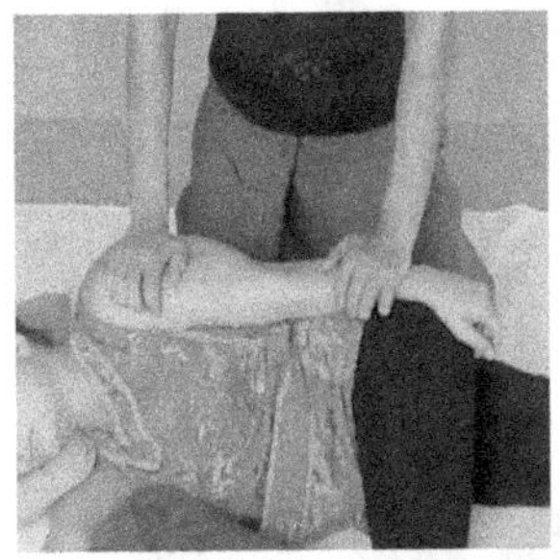

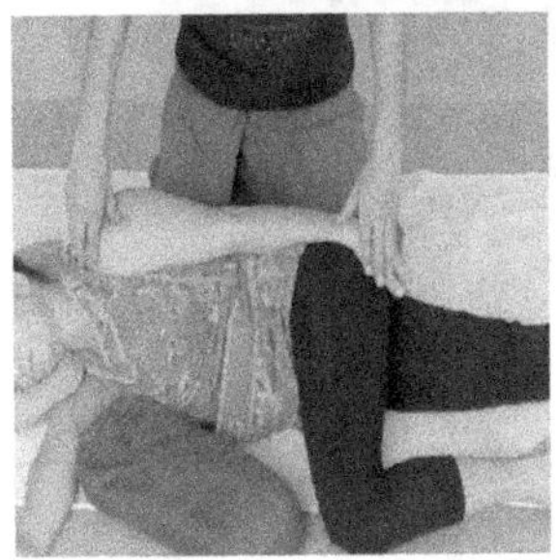

6-Thumb walk + palm walk.

We perform a thumb walk, from the outside in, between the ulna and radius on the forearm, and over the line of the humerus on the upper arm. We then repeat the Palmer walk. Be careful when performing the thumb pressure on the arm, remember that the pressure is going in the direction of the humerus, and it can cause pain.

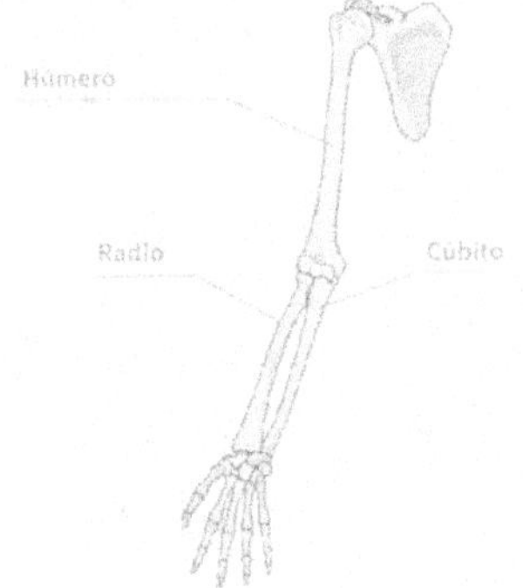

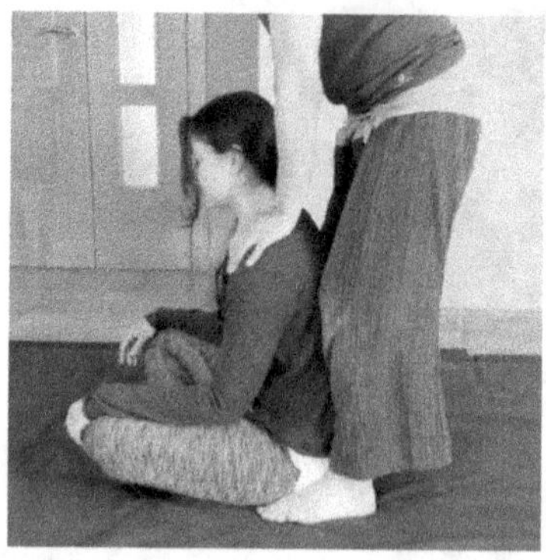

7-Change position + sitting position.

We ask the client to turn to the other side and repeat techniques 1 through 7. We then help the client move to the seated position, passing behind the back while performing alternating Palm pressure on the trapezius. This will help relieve tension and upper back pain. If the client is unable to maintain their posture, you can try asking them to stretch their legs or place a cushion or zafu behind them and ask them to sit on it.

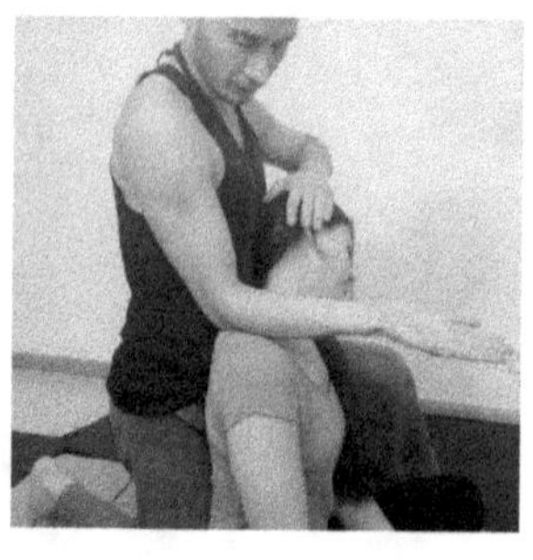

8-THE ROLLING PIN TECHNIQUE.

We guide the c'lients head to one side and hold it with our hand or forearm. With the other forearm we perform a forward roll only. The starting point is with the palm down, then we roll the forearm and the hand ends upward. The movement is always forward -- that is, you should roll the arm forward two or three times, then start again from the starting point. The rolling pin helps to relieve tension without having to use your hands. Repeat on the other side and then center the head and perform the technique with both forearms at the same time.

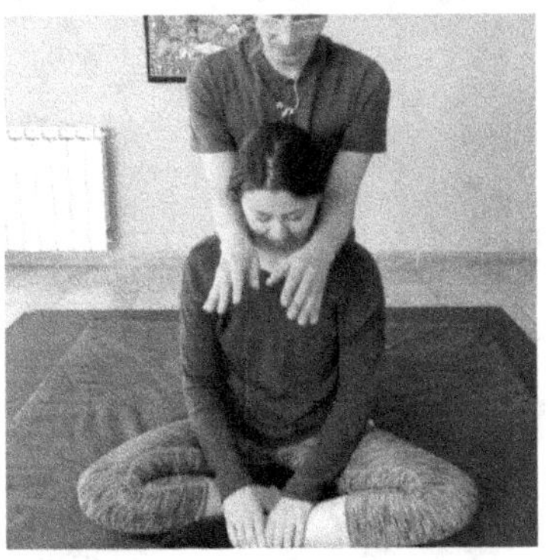

9-Stretching + walking the back.

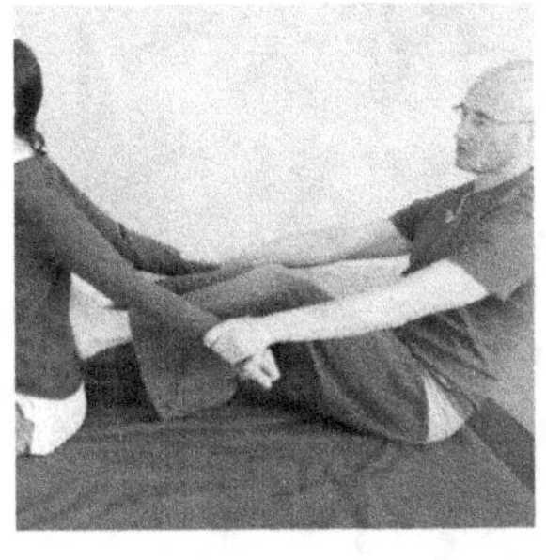

We take her hands and bring them back, sit down and place your feet in the scapular area and perform a stretching by taking her arms backwards. We repeat, this time with our feet two or three thumbs down. Then we start walking the back down and up several times. This helps to release tension on the entire back, also opens the chest and shoulders, and improves spinal alignment.

10- Torsion.

We place the client's hands behind the neck and instruct them to interlace the fingers. We stand up, take the elbows and place the outside part of our leg on the client's back. We ask the client to inhale deeply, then tell her to exhale and as she does so, we guide the client's body into a twist. We must be attentive to body's resistance.

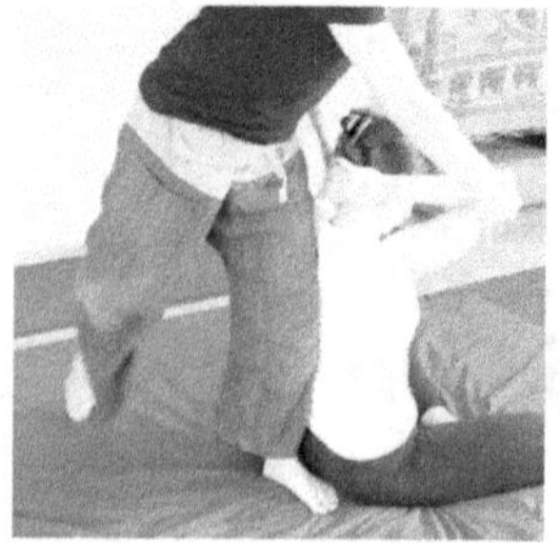

You have to be very careful in the case of a lumbar injury. This is a great stretch for the back, especially the lower back.

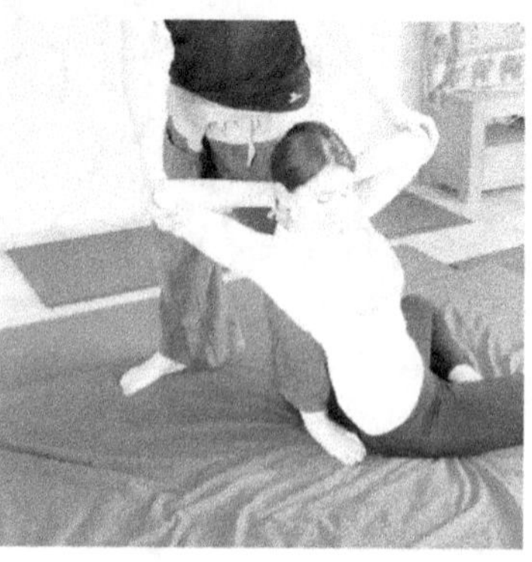

11-Nut cracker.

We move the client's head forward to better expose the cervical area. We interlace our fingers and perform a compression with both of our hands on three points of the neck, moving up and down with moderate pressure. Ask the client how the pressure feels and adjust accord-

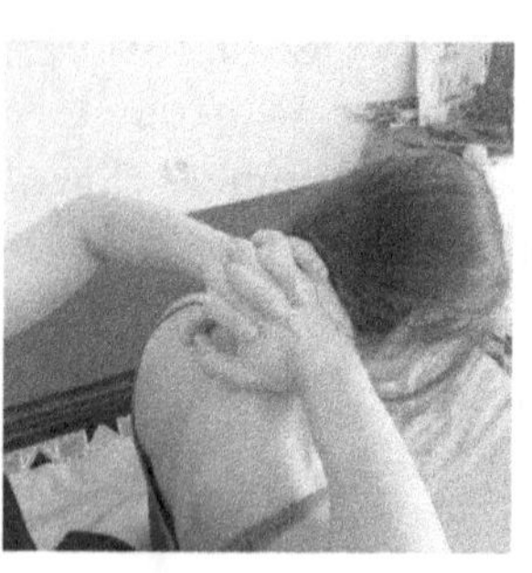

ingly. This technique is excellent for relieving neck pain. It also helps in cases of headache, stress, insomnia and lack of concentration.

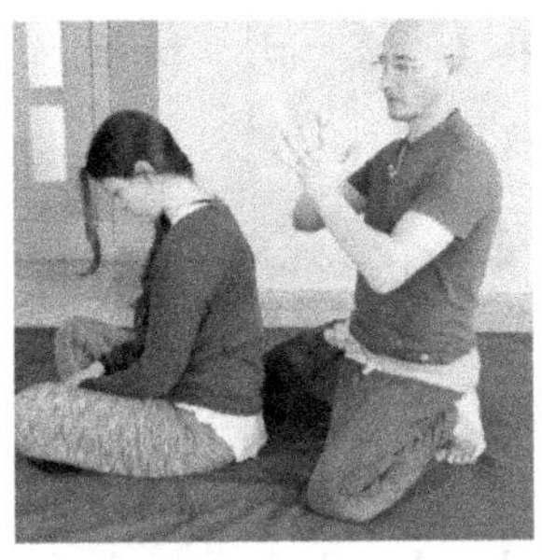

12-THAI PERCUSSION.

Join hands together, hands open, elbows open and wrists loose. We move our hands back and forth, percussing the entire upper back. Make sure your wrists are moving and not your arms. It should be a fluid movement. Check out the free videos on learnthaimassage.net/videoguide.

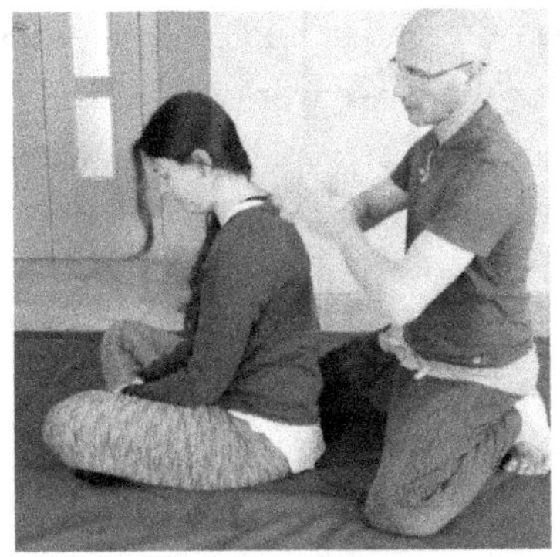

13-Sweeping and final contact.

We make a sweep with both hands on the back, ending with a final contact. You can put your hands together wherever you feel relevant, but I usually do it just above the spine, at the level of the shoulder blades. Then you move in front of the client

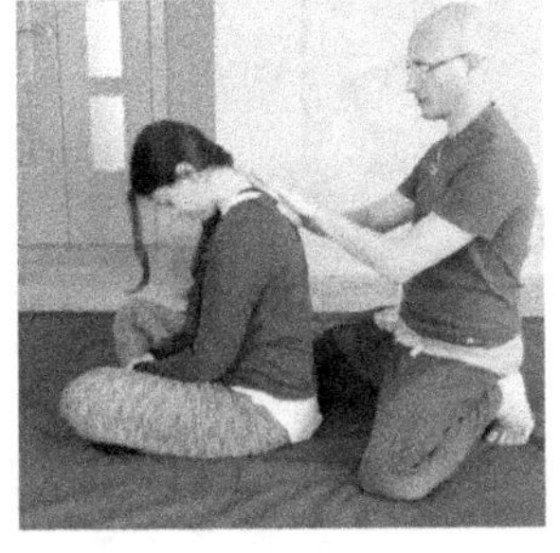

and with your hands together you bow as a form of gratitude for having had the opportunity to offer the message session.

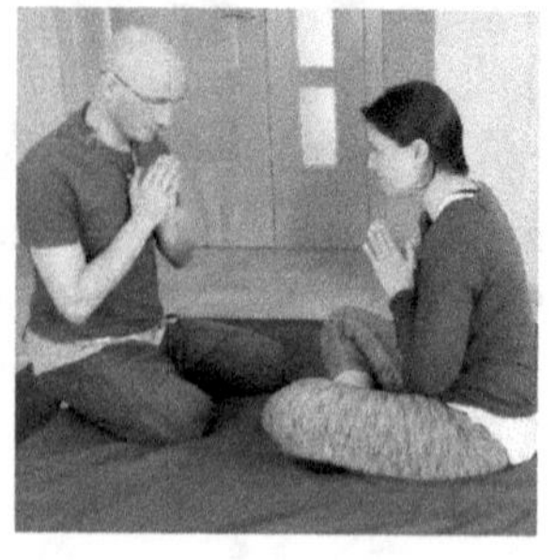

From there, you should allow a few moments for the client to return to normal state. When they do so, I recommend that you ask for feedback, that is, that you ask them how they have felt throughout the massage session, if they feel more relieved and/or with more pain in any area of the body and also that they describe that pain. Many times when we work on muscle tension, we can leave a sensation of pain, a pain different from that of the tension itself, a pain that at the same time feels good, so it is convenient that we communicate with the client to see what kind of pain it is if she feels any.

CHAPTER 10
THAI MASSAGE ON A TABLE

When I started working on cruise ships, I ran into a problem. Even though I loved the job, they wouldn't let me do Thai massages because it wasn't part of the spa protocol. I knew that if I didn't somehow manage to practice, I would lose my skill set. So to stop this from happening, I came up with two things:

The first thing I did was do a Thai massage for my colleagues after work. This left me exhausted from working long hours, but it brought me many friends.

The second thing that occurred to me was doing a Thai massage during my working hours, and adapting it to the massage table. I was given carte blanche to include some acupressure and assisted stretching, so as long as I complied with the minimum spa protocol and what the client requested, I could do more or less whatever I wanted.

I included some versions of traditional techniques and on some occasions I did a free adaptation so that Thai techniques could fit well with the spa protocols on the table.

Below I am going to show some very simple techniques

so that you begin to realize that the scope of Thai technique goes beyond what you can do on the floor. If you want to go deeper and see the result of my experiments when I was working in spas, there's more in my book "Thai Massage on a table".

PRONE POSITION:

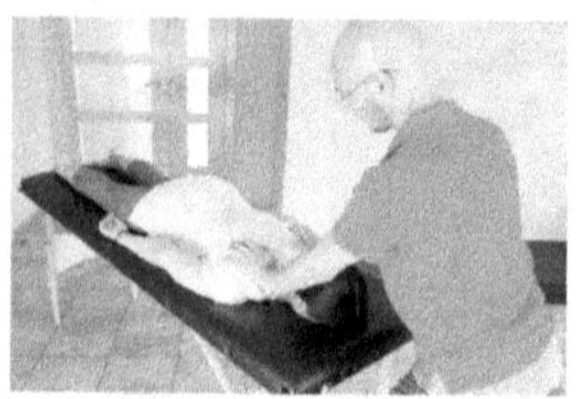

1- Palmar pressure on trapezius.

We simply stand behind the client's head, and do an alternating palmar pressure on the trapezius, as if we were walking in place, apply pressure on the heels of the hands. Take the opportunity to observe the level of tension in that part of the back.

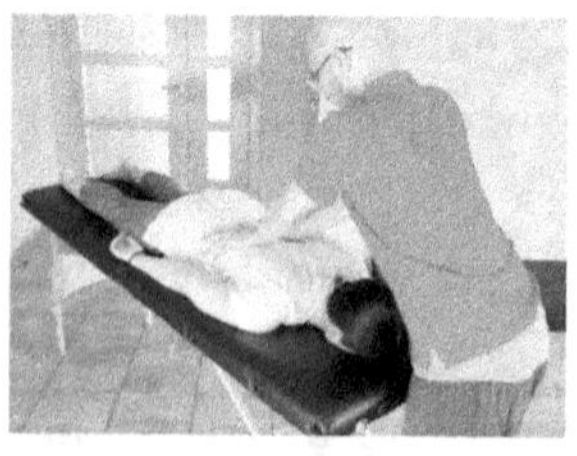

2-PALM WALK ALONG THE BACK.

We walk with our palms from the trapezius to the lumbar area back and forth. You can repeat multiple times until you feel that the tension is giving way.

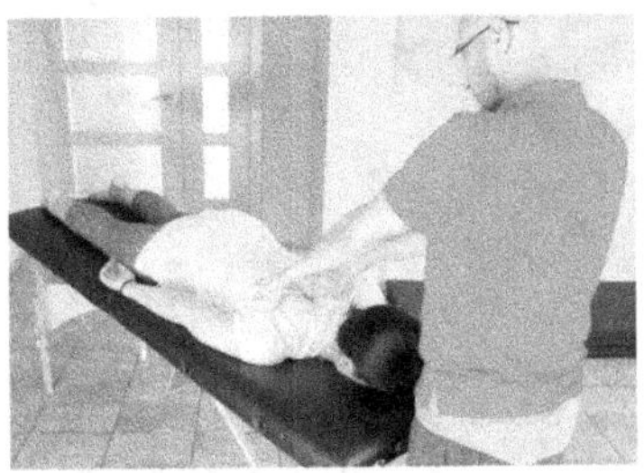

3-THUMB WALK.

In the same way that we worked lines 1 and 2 on the floor, we're going to do the same from here. We press with the pads of our thumbs, 6 to 8 points along line 1 (between spine and paravertebral) and line 2 (above the paravertebral).

4-PALM WALK AGAIN.

We again do a palmar walk along the back, to soften the sensation left by the line work with the thumbs.

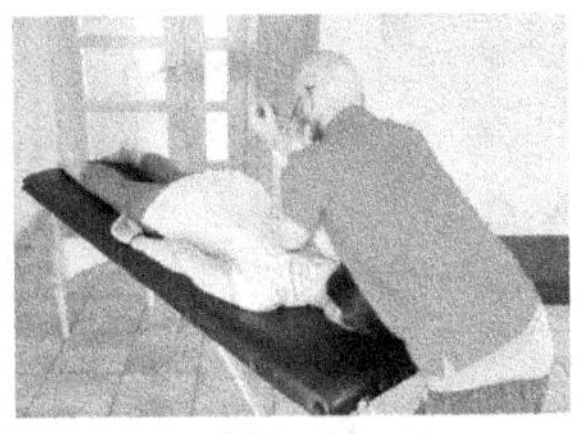

5-Elbows.

Here we make an alternating pressure with elbows in two positions. First, touch the tip of the scapula and the upper edge of the scapula. Once you iden-tify the first two parts, draw an imaginary line down the middle. The first point is on this line and the second point is two fingers below it. I am talking about bilateral points -- that is, you are going to work on one side and the other side of the spine. Pressure has to be done with the tip of the elbow.

. . .

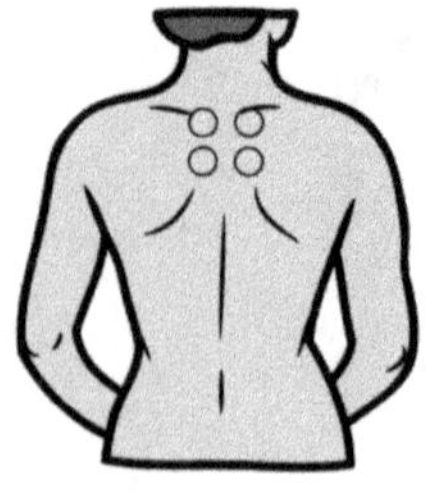

6-PRESSURE POINTS.

You have to go gradually because they are usually sensitive points but at the same time pleasant for the client. They are often called "hungry points" because although they hurt, they need pressure and they are the ones that with the right pressure, the client usually says "it hurts but I like it". Apply pressure to these points until you feel some relief and muscle decompression.

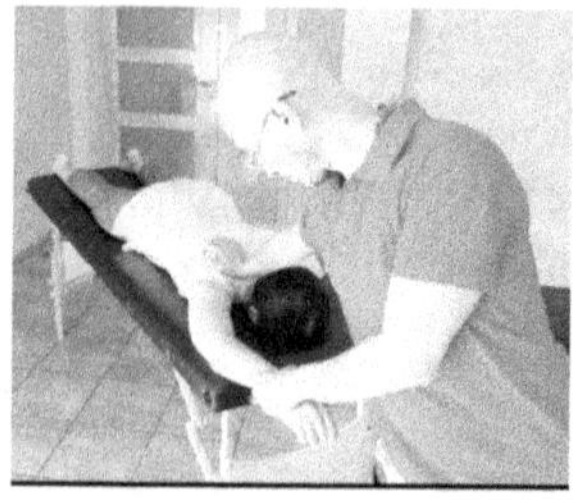

7-PRESSURE AND STRETCHING.

Now we stretch the arm above the head, and while stretching the wrist, we perform a compression with the palm on the trapezius area. In this way we relieve tension and at the same time stretch the arm, shoulder and dorsal torso. Repeat with the other arm.

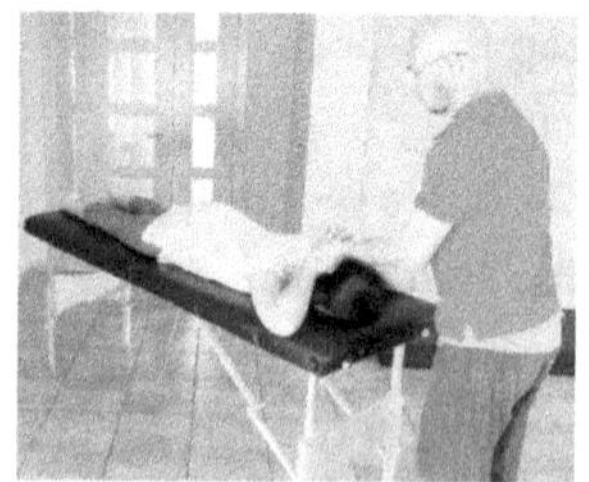

8-EXTENSION (PREPARATION I)..

Now we are going to do a chest opening. To do this, the first step is to bring both hands of the client behind their neck and ask them to interlace their fingers.

. . .

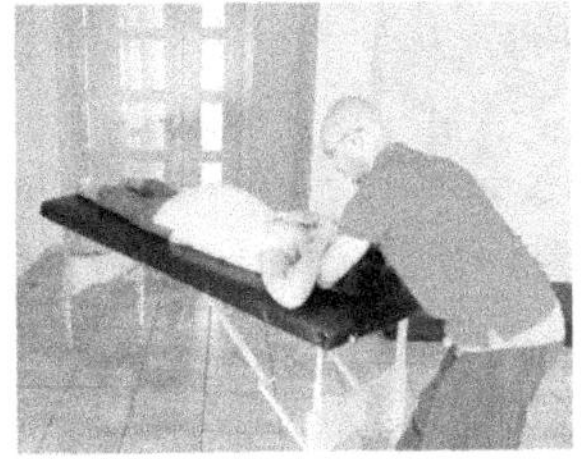

9-EXTENSION (PREPARATION 2).

We pass our arms down under the client's forearms and place our hands together behind their back, forming an inverted "V".

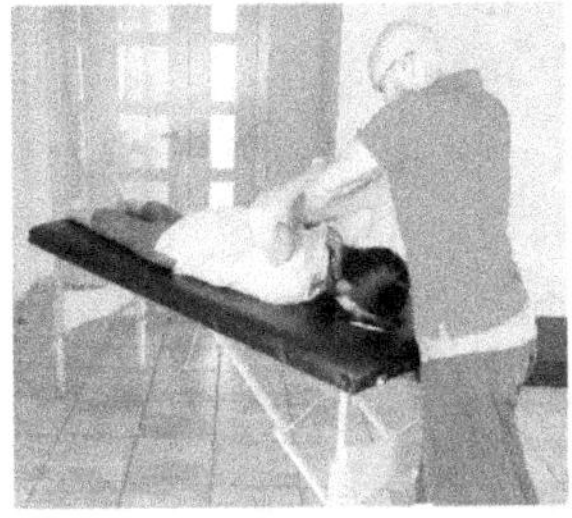

10-EXTENSION.

We lift our bodies and extend our arms to bring the elbows of the client backwards and thus create a chest extension. Note, that the model has a lot of flexibility, so the body does not lift too much, but with a person with less elasticity the movement will be more noticeable.

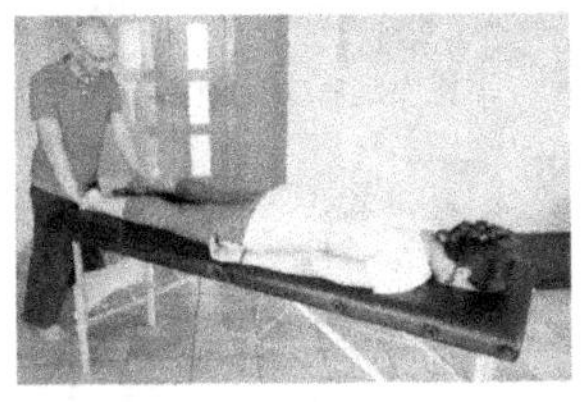

11-PALM PRESSURE ON THE FEET.

Now we go to the feet and perform alternating pressure with the palms on the feet. The pressure is on the soles, and you can put a slight outward pressure on the heels if there is not much resistance.

11-PALM WALK ON THE LEGS.

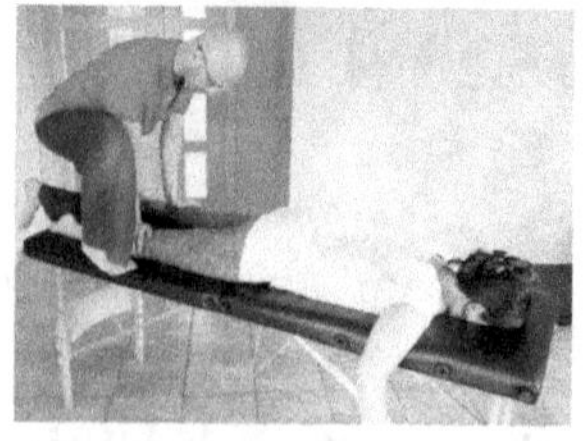

We climb onto the massage table with one knee between the client's legs, in a warrior position, or kneeling with both knees between the client's feet. We do a Palmar walk on two points in the calf area and two points in the hamstring area.

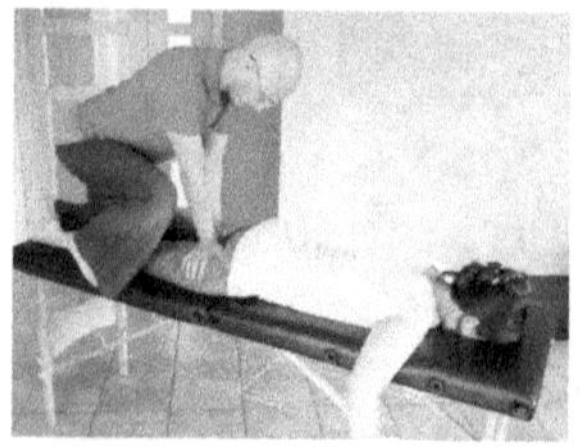

11B-PALM WALK ON THE LEGS.

We go up to the gluteal line and back again. As long as you feel comfortable, you can take a few walks. In fact, it is recommended that you do it if the person has circulation problems or a lot of tension in the legs.

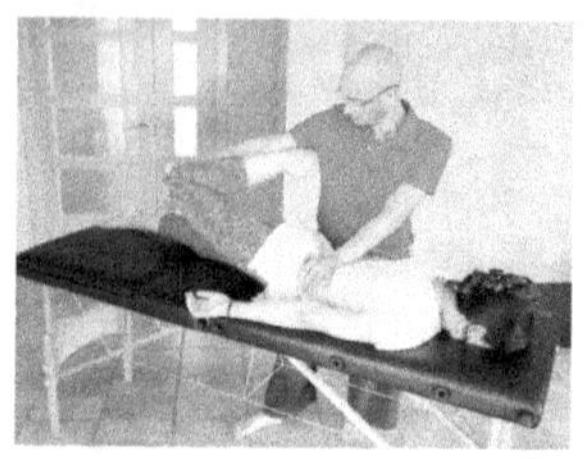

12-LEG STRETCHING.

We look for the opposite leg and bring the client's foot under our armpit. We hold the knee with one hand and our other hand rests on the lumbar area, while the receiver's foot goes under our armpit. Now we lift the knee and put pressure on the lower back. Here we stretch the quadriceps, open the hips, and decompress the lower back.

13-ELBOW PRESSURE ON THE BUTTOCKS..

We apply pressure with the elbow in the center of the

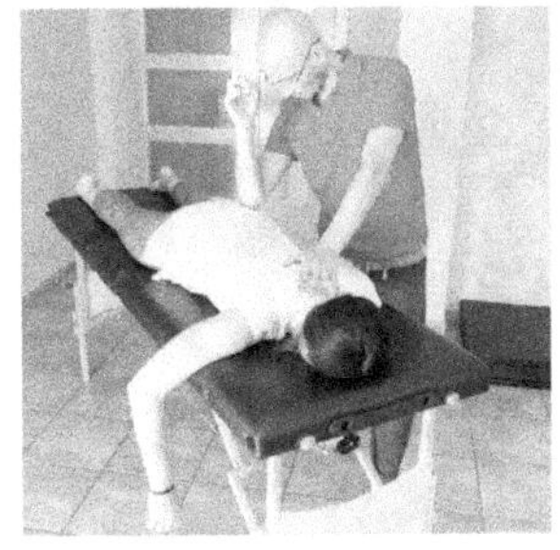

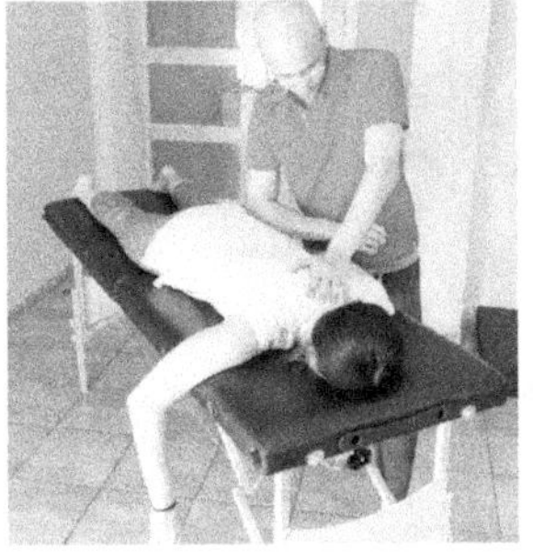

buttock. Right in this area you will find a small depression, this is especially good for treating lower back pain and sciatic pain. Be sure to go with gradual pressure as it is usually painful.

13b- Pressure with forearm on buttocks.

For some people the pressure with the elbow may be too strong, in these cases it is convenient that the work is done with the forearm, you can also alternate pressure with the elbow and forearm.

SUPINE POSITION:

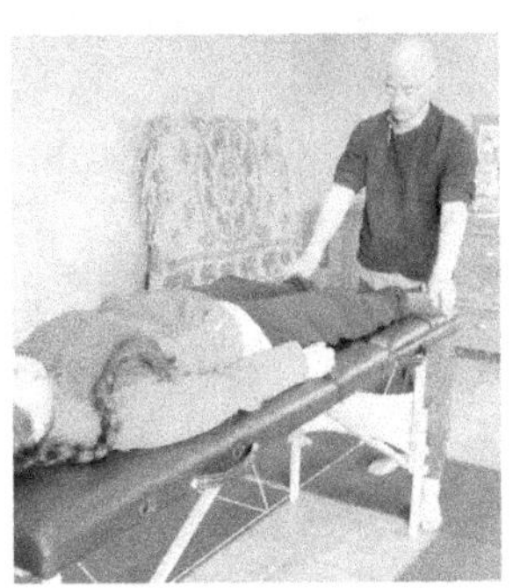

1-Thumb walk on the feet.

We are going to do a thumb walk over the arch line of the feet, back and forth several times.

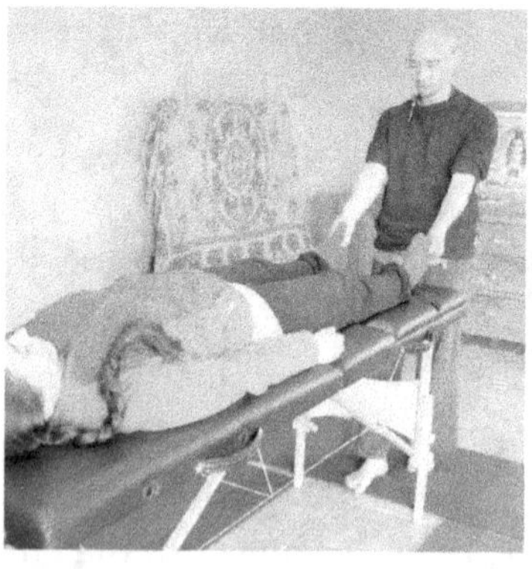

2-FINGER ROTATION AND STRETCHING.

We will take each finger from the base and make three rotations to one side and three to the other. Then we stretch well.

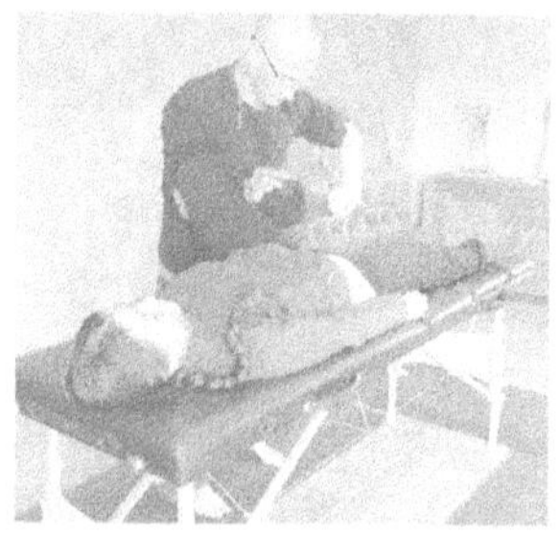

3-COMPOUND MANEUVER.

Lift the leg up and bend it. Place the forearm under the knee, close to the popliteal fossa. We bring the knee of the client towards the chest and put pressure on the instep, as if trying to bring the heel down to the buttock. This technique stretches the lower back, stimulates the hamstrings and calves, and decompresses the knee.

4-DA KU KHA adapted to the table.

We place the client's foot on our hip and then hold the knee. Our other hand puts pressure on three points on the opposite leg (groin area, medial and 4 toes above the knee)

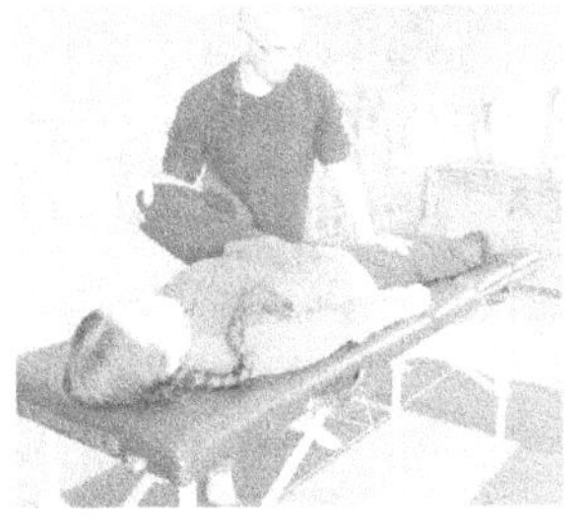

while at the same time we rock forward and backward to bring the knee forward to stretch the lumbar spine. Repeat the 4 and 5 on the other side.

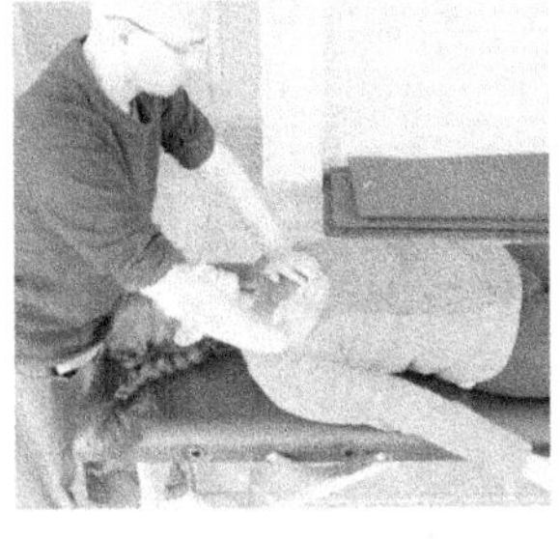

5-PALMAR PRESSURE ON PECTORALS.

We place ourselves behind the head of the client, with our hands forming an upside down "V," creating an alternating palmar pressure on the upper pectoral. This is a simple technique that gives a great feeling of relaxation, but if the person has big boobs, we must be careful not to be too invasive and that the person feels comfortable.

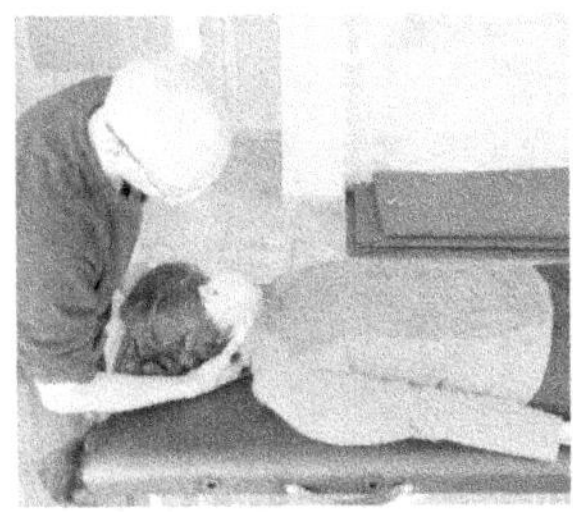

6-NECK MASSAGE.

Turn the head to one side and apply circular pressure with your thumb, index or index plus middle finger. Loosen the tension and switch to the other side.

7-STRETCHING AND COMPRESSION.

We bring the arm above the head by holding it against

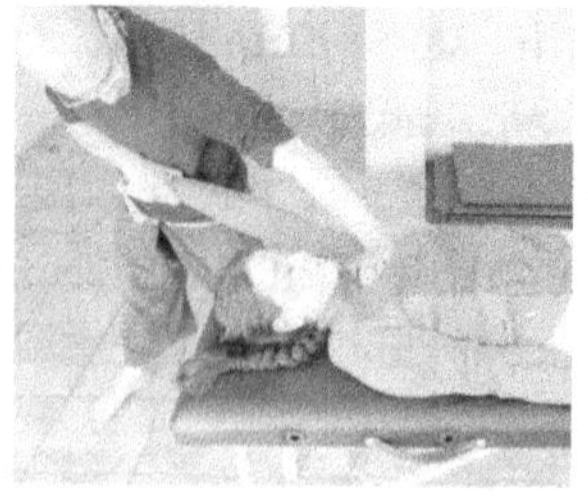

the wrist. The other hand is on the pectoral. Apply pressure on the pectoral while stretching the arm.

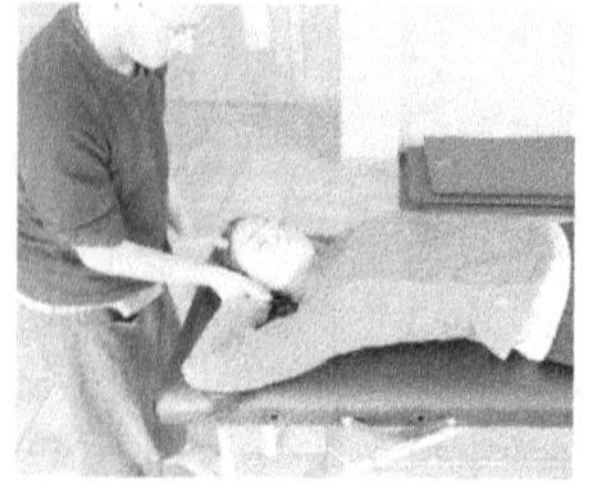

8-THE KETTLE (PREPARATION).

We place the client's hand over his ear (Note: here it would be more appropriate to continue on the same side where we did the last maneuver, I have decided to show the image from the opposite side for a matter of visual clarity).

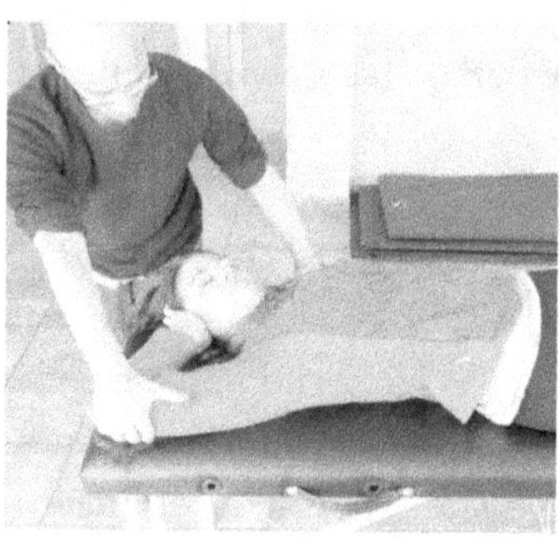

8-THE KETTLE (STARTING POINT).

Now we place one hand on the client's elbow and the other on the opposite shoulder.

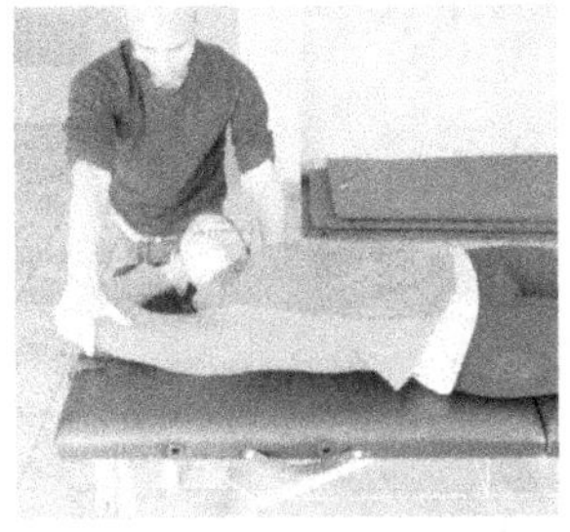

8B- THE KETTLE (STRETCHING).

Using our body, we pull the elbow back while applying pressure on the shoulder. Here we are stretching the cervical, triceps and dorsal while compressing the shoulders. We repeat on the other side: 7 and 8.

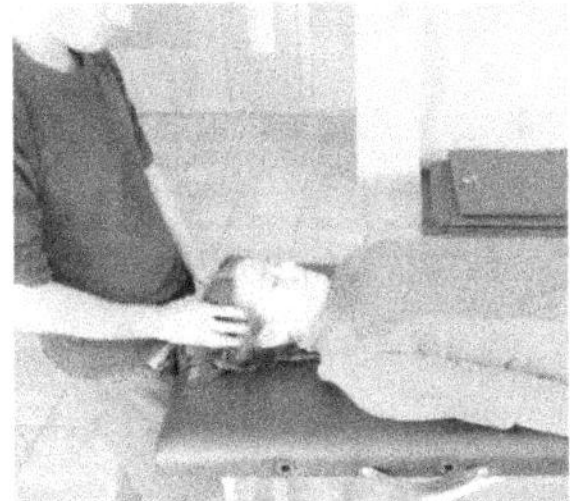

9-SCALP MASSAGE.

Finish with a circular pressure with the fingers over the entire scalp. It is important to maintain a calm rhythm. We use this technique to facilitate relaxation.

IF YOU LIKED this simplified Thai massage routine adapted to the table, you will find a much more in the upcoming book Thai Massage on a Table.

CHAPTER 11
THAI MASSAGE WITH
THE FEET

Working with the feet has been one of the best skills I have been able to learn. Not only do you offer a different sensation to the client, doing foot massage allows you to take the strain off your back, arms and hands. You can exert significant pressure and relieve tension with minimal effort even with very large bodies.

Below I will introduce you to some basic back massage techniques so that you can begin to include them in your therapies.

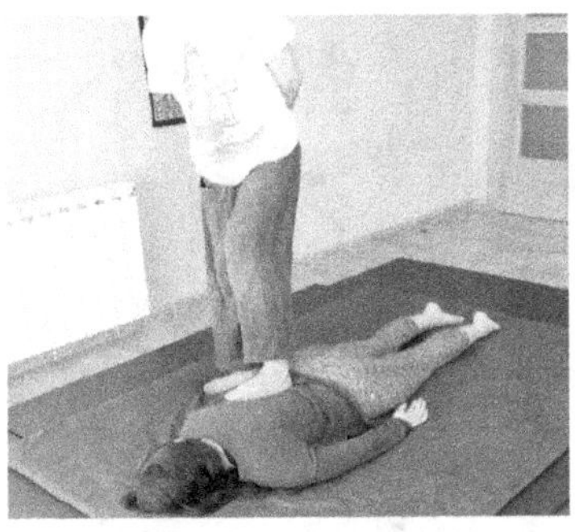

1-SIMPLE PRESSURE: position 1.

With the client in the prone position, we place ourselves on the side of the back and raise one foot up. We place it on the lumbar area, right above the sacrum. We apply pressure through the heel.

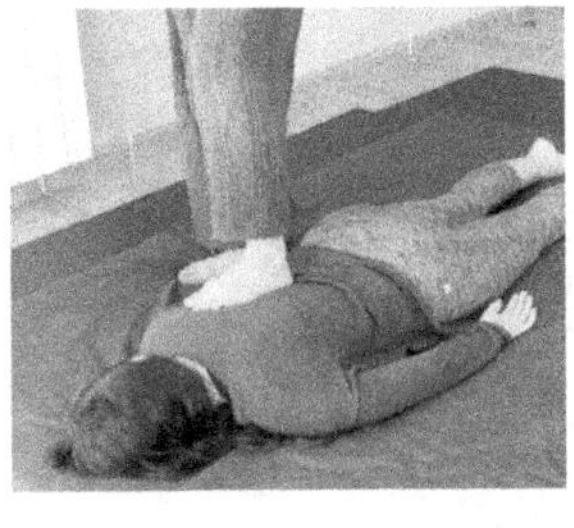

2-SIMPLE PRESSURE: position 2.

The second pressure is in the dorsal area, always next to the spine (on our side). The tip of our foot is just a little forward of the lower edge of the scapula. Here we can distribute the pressure between the heel and the metatarsus.

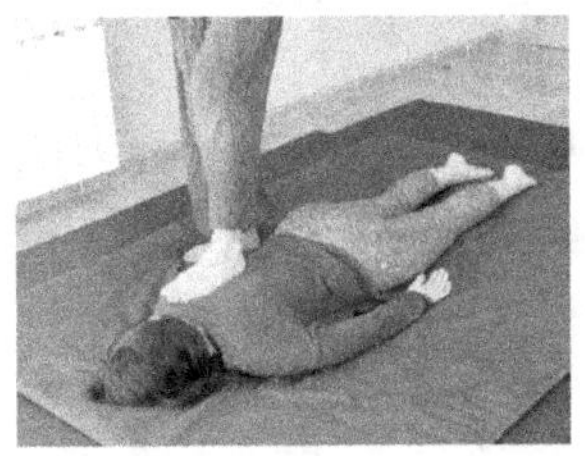

3-Simple pressure: position 3.

We advance a little more with the foot, and this time the tip of the foot remains on the upper edge of the scapula.

. . .

LET'S review the positions of the feet in these drawings.

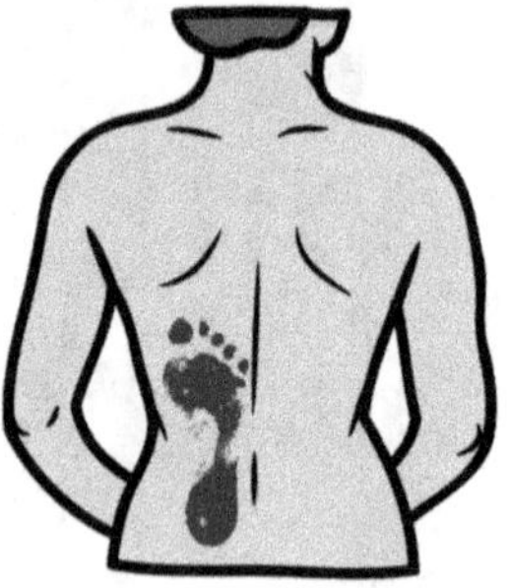

Position 1: Remember that the position of your toes will depend on the size of the client.

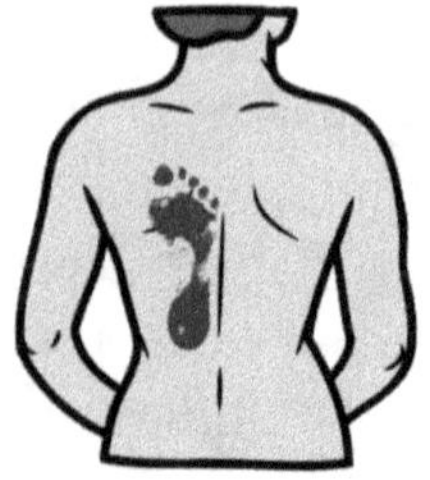

POSITION 2: You can now focus the pressure on the outer edge of your foot, so that it compresses and stimulates the paravertebrals.

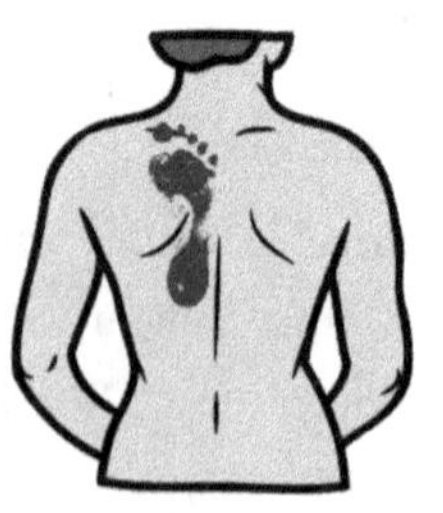

IDEALLY, when we press the left side of the back, the client should head to the right, and when we press the right side, the head should face to the left. The pressure is gradual, deep, and slow. Work back and forth several times until you begin to feel the back loosen. It is very important and helpful to ask the receiver how they are receiving it. If you find it difficult to maintain stability, you can use a cane or a chair.

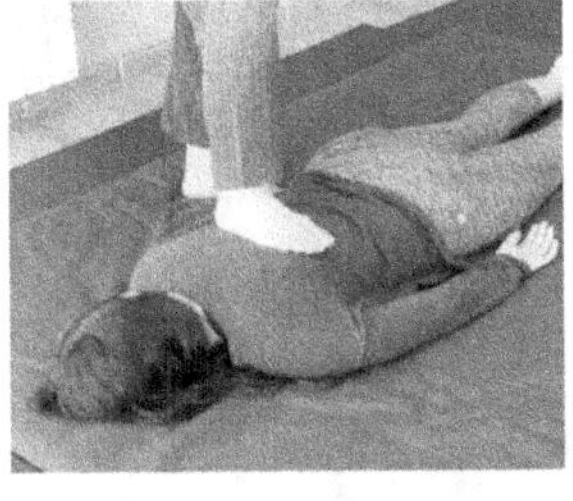

4-CROSSED FOOT PRESSURE 1.

Now we are going to cross the spine with a foot. Don't worry, as most of the pressure will be concentrated on the heel and metatarsus, and it will not adversely affect the vertebrae. The foot goes through the scapular area, over the lower part of the scapula.

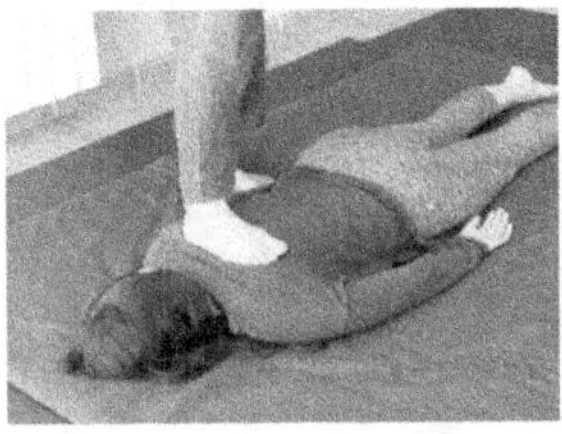

5-CROSSED FOOT PRESSURE 2.

We advance with the foot to the upper edge of the shoulder blades and unload the weight gradually. We alternate between these two points back and forth several times.

REVIEW OF CROSSED FOOT POSITIONS.

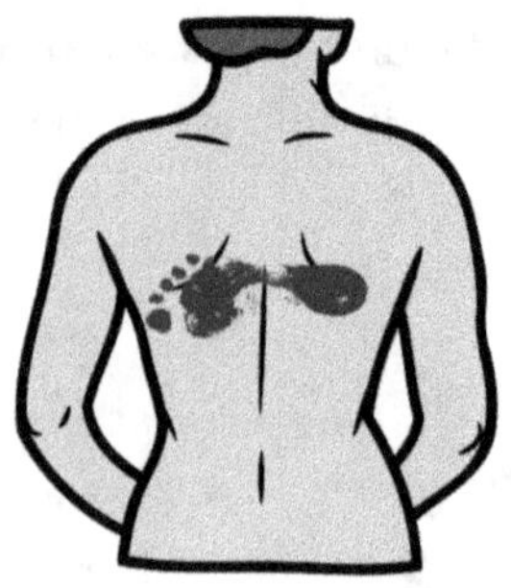

POSITION 1.

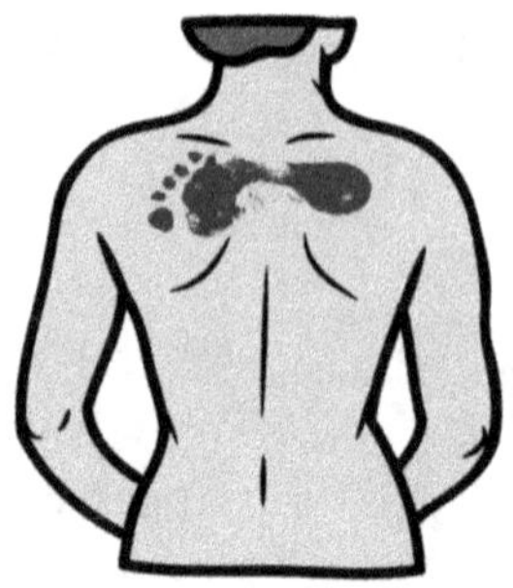

POSITION 2.

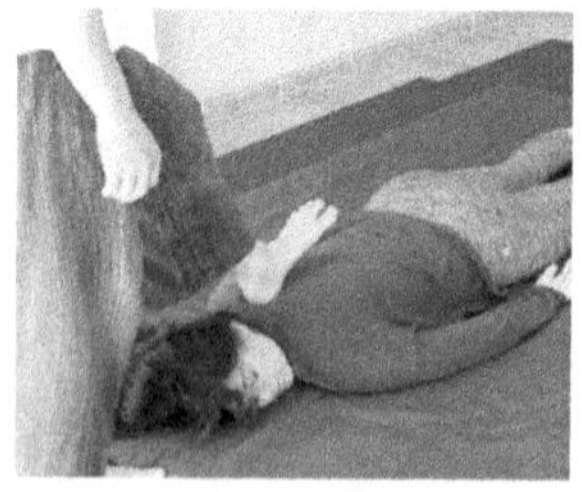

6-HEEL on upper back (trapezius muscle).

Here we also have to make sure that the client is facing away from where we are pressing. The points are next to the spine on the line of the middle of the scapulae and on the line of the upper edge of the scapulae.

. . .

Upper back points review.

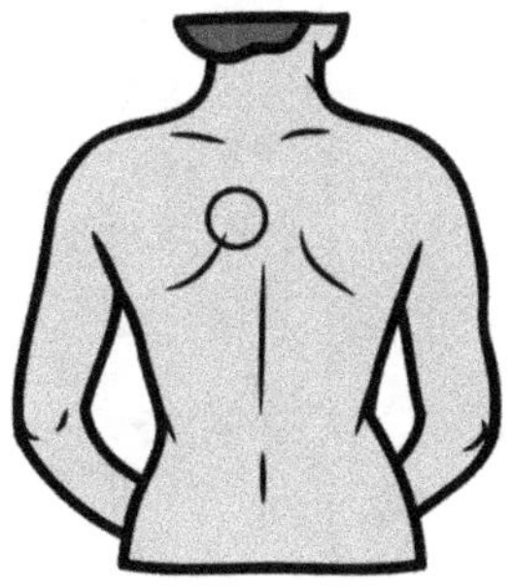

Point 1.

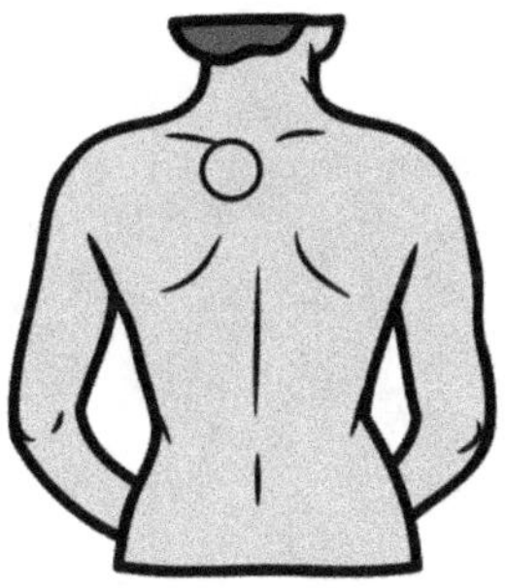

Point 2.

These points require strong pressure. It is important that you do not lose stability in order to exert intense but gradual pressure at the same time.

. . .

THIS SIMPLE ROUTINE will help you become familiar with using your feet as a therapeutic tool. When you use your feet, you will see a big difference in your energy and hands. Plus, clients will love it.

CHAPTER 12
THAI ABDOMINAL MASSAGE

Although I have already included abdominal massage in this book, I have decided to add this chapter to expand a little more and also because:

1-It is a rather neglected subject in Thai massage courses.

2-The technique is relatively simple.

3-The benefits are great.

To begin with, abdominal massage is much more therapeutic than you might imagine. Working on the abdomen activates very important functions in the body, such as blood and lymph circulation, digestive, respiratory, renal, and sexual function. In Thai medicine, organs are associated with emotions and the energy of the elements.

The following is a list of the main organs and their relationship within the framework of traditional Thai medicine:

LIVER:

Emotion: anger.

Element: fire.

. . .

KIDNEYS AND LUNGS:
Emotion: sadness.
Element: water.

HEART:
Emotion: happiness.
Element: fire.

KIDNEYS[1]:
Emotion: fear.
Element: water.

STOMACH AND INTESTINES:
Emotion: worry.
Element: wind.

THIS MEANS that an organ condition can lead to an imbalance on an energetic and emotional level, and at the same time, an internal organ massage can bring benefits in both directions as well.

That is to say that abdominal massage should be included to positively affect the function of internal organs, energy balance, and emotional balance, and there is an additional benefit that needs to be included: help to reduce imbalances in the lower back.

Sometimes lower back pain can come from a problem in the viscera, so abdominal massage completes the therapeutic work when we need an emphasis on the lumbar area of the body. In other words, if the client is experiencing lower back pain, a good way to help him would be to do a good massage in the lumbar area, some reflexology work (for example working feet and ears) and spending a portion of the session in the abdomen.

Now we will see the techniques, if you want to learn more, check the thai abdominal massage online course at shivathai.net.

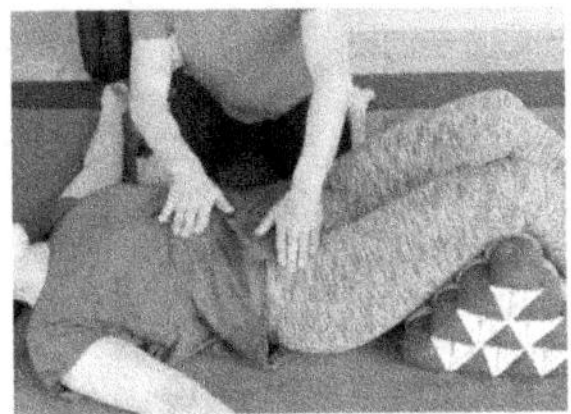

1-Circular friction.

Preferably, we place the legs on a cushion and then elevate them. We now perform circular friction in a clockwise direction.

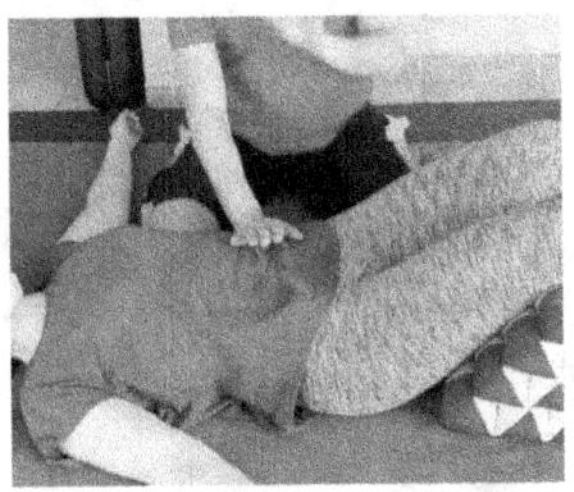

2-THE WAVE (PREPARATION).

We place the heel of the hand where the obliques fall, on our side.

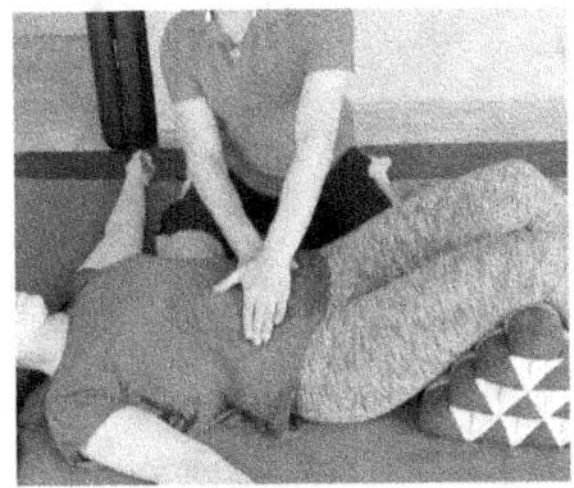

2-THE WAVE (PREPARATION).

Place the other hand on top and then slightly further. The fingertips should be on the oblique side of the opposite side. The hands should be supported and relaxed.

. . .

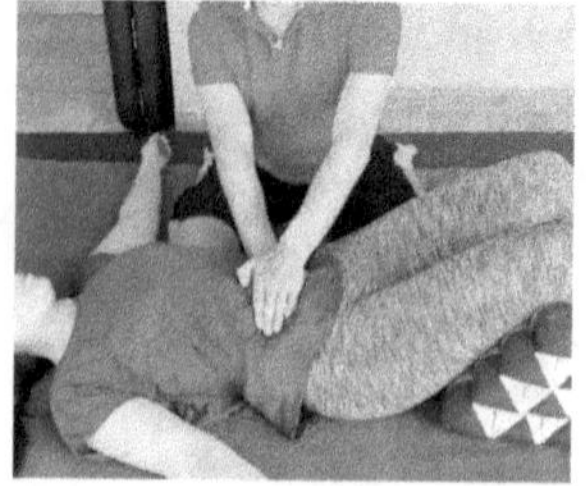

2-THE WAVE (PUSH).

From here, we make an inward and forward pressure, as if we wanted to push internal organs.

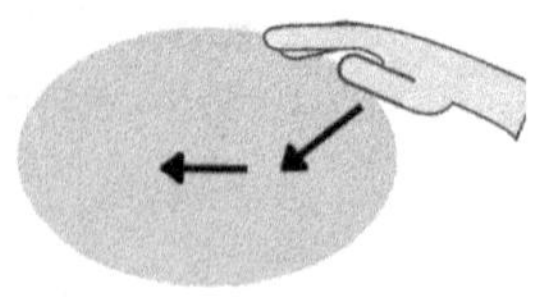

2-THE WAVE (PUSH).

Here I am showing you the direction of pressure, inward and forward. It is not sliding, it is compression. If you feel friction in the palm, that means you are sliding, what you should notice is tissue movement.

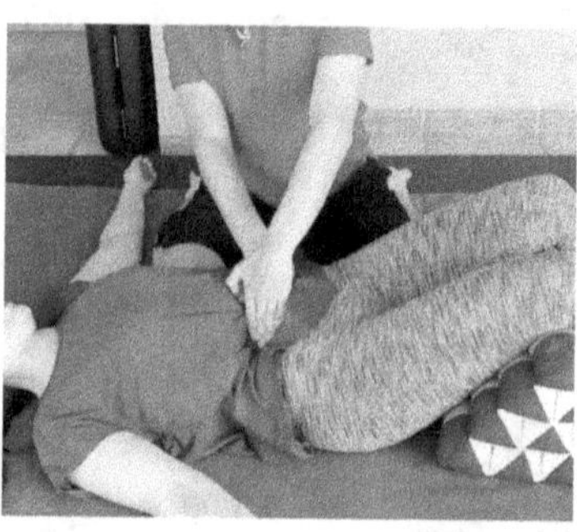

2-The wave (pull).

Here, to do the opposite movement, you have to pull, that is, push as much tissue as you can with your fingertips in your direction, like a returning wave.

. . .

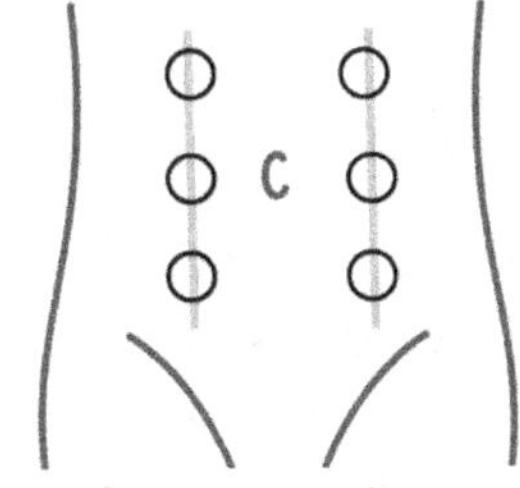

3-ACUPRESSURE POINTS.

To locate the points we need to identify the navel, this is our reference point. Now we are going to measure two fingers on each side of the navel and mentally draw a vertical line along each side of the navel. From here, two fingers above the navel are the first two pressure points. At navel level there are two points. Two fingers below the navel is the third pair of points. Keep in mind that when you measure with your fingers, the correct measurement is the client's fingers, so if there is too much difference in physique between you and the client, you will have to adjust this distance.

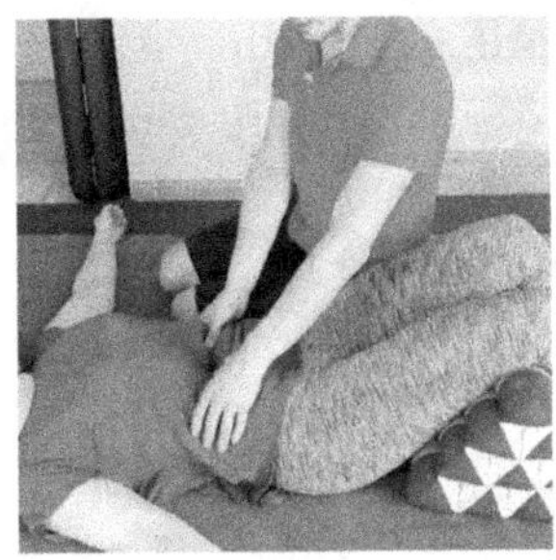

3-Acupressure.

Let's apply thumb pressure on three bilateral points. We place our fingers on the first pair of points, ask the receiver to inhale, and when we tell him to exhale, we enter with a simultaneous, gradual and deep pressure there. When he inhales again, we release the pressure and continue with the other points. We continue with point 2 (navel line) and 3 (two fingers below the navel), and return to point 2 and finally point 1. If the receiver is too sensitive, lower the intensity to a pressure it can tolerate.

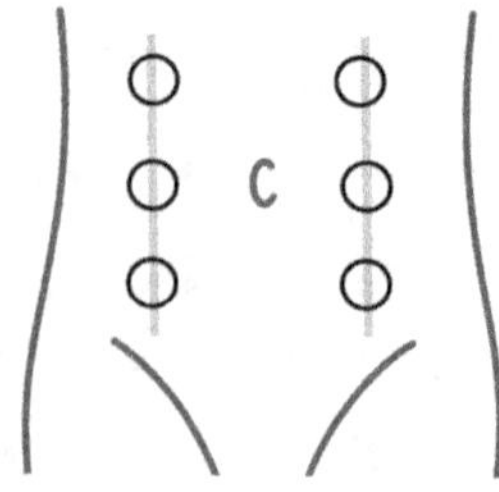

4-Acupressure 2.

Measure 4 fingers on each side of the navel and repeat the steps above. It is useful to mark the inhalation and exhalation as noises. That is, when you inhale you compress the glottis, and when you exhale you release the air through the mouth making the sound "shhh" as though you're asking for silence. This is useful when the client is too relaxed, when he or she does not know how to take a deep breath, and when he or she is in a lot of pain.

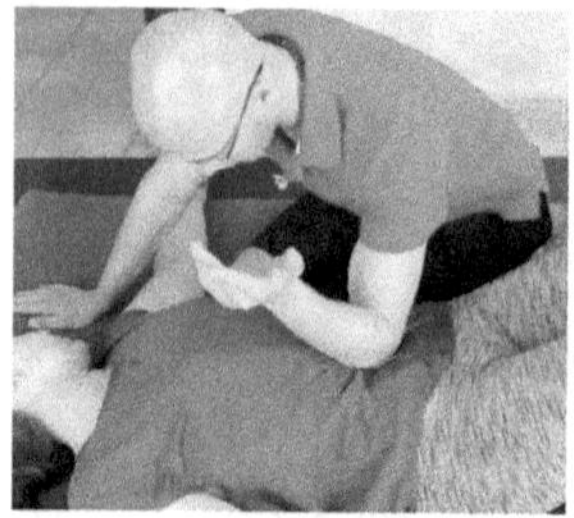

4-PRESSURE ON THE NAVEL.

We place the elbow on the navel and when the receiver exhales we apply pressure. We maintain this pressure for as long as possible for 4 respiratory cycles and then we slowly release the pressure.

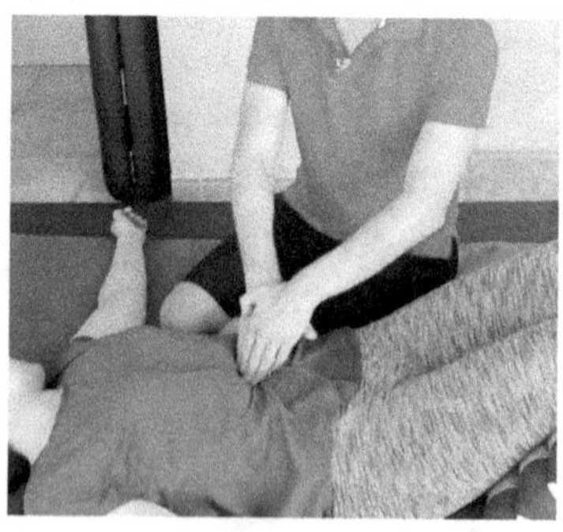

5-PRESSURE on 6 points vertical line.

We put our hands together and with our fingertips we exert pressure on points 1 through 6 back and forth. As always, the pressure should be gradual and deep. You can simply press or make a small circle when entering deep.

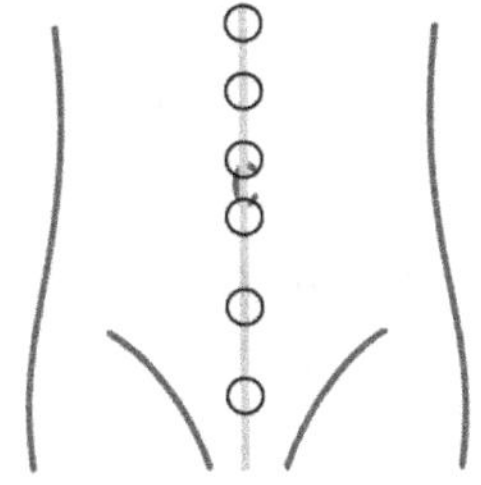

5-LOCATION OF POINTS.

The first point is two fingers below the xiphoid process, the tip of the sternum. The second point is between the first point and the upper edge of the navel. The third point is at the upper edge of the navel. The fourth point is at the lower edge of the navel. The fifth point is between points 4 and 6. The sixth point is one finger above the pubic bone.

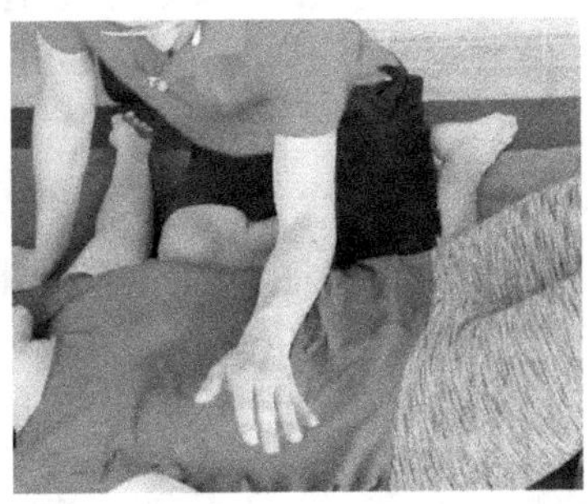

6-THE ROLLER (INITIAL POSITION).

Here's what we're going to do: forearm roll pressure. We place the forearm across the abdomen, below the ribs with the palm facing down.

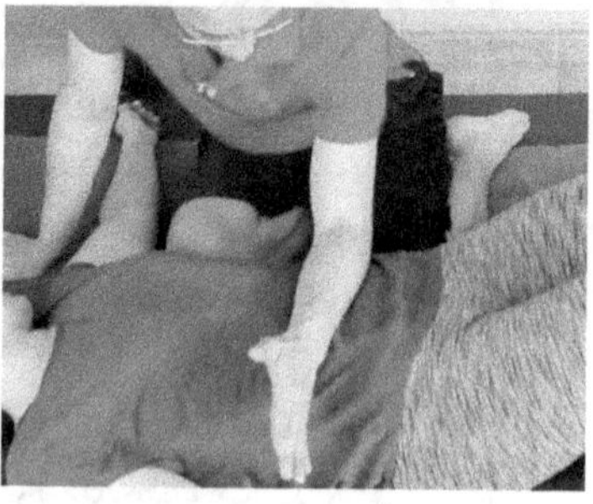

6-The roller (intermediate position).

We begin to roll the forearm while exerting gentle pressure with the forearm.

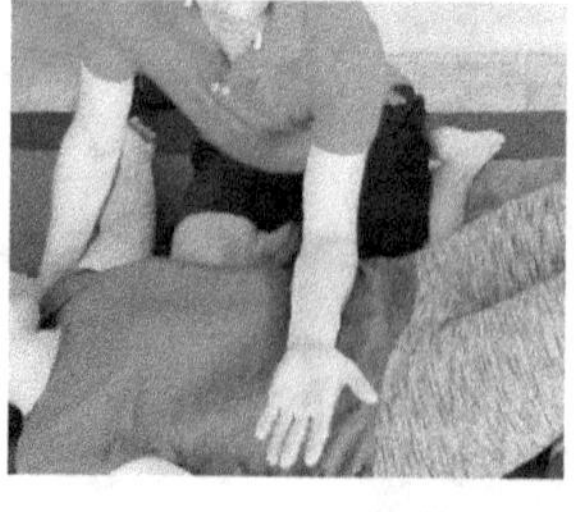

6-THE ROLLER (FINAL POSITION).

We finish rolling the forearm, keeping the palm pointing upward. The forearm would be more or less at the level of the navel. From here we move the palm downward and roll the forearm one or two more times until it reaches the end of the abdomen.

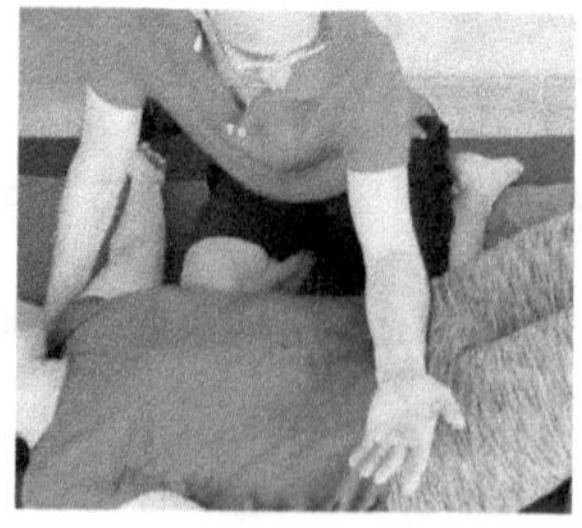

6-THE ROLLER (until the end of the abdomen area).

Here we see how we reach the end of the abdomen. Once here, we return the forearm to the initial position under the ribs and repeat. The sensation should be like that of a rolling pin, going from top to bottom several times.

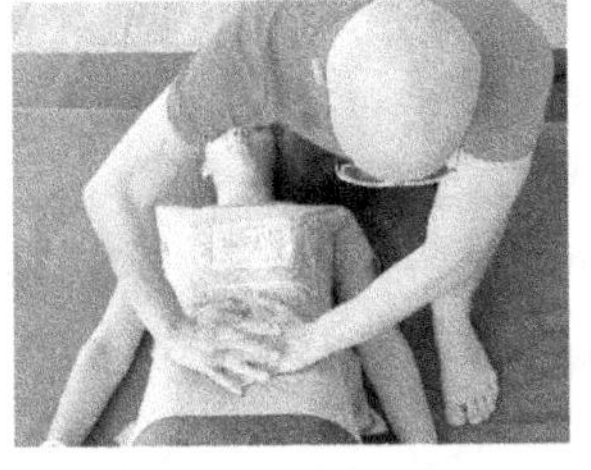

7-OSTEOTHAI.

Now I want to show you an osteothai maneuver, a technique developed by the French master David Lutt. Facing in the direction of the client's feet, we interlace our fingers and make a double wave. That is, pressure to one side and to the other, but this time very gentle. There is no sliding, just a relaxed movement, as if we were moving through water. Unlike the previous ones, this is a very subtle and superficial maneuver, but it has a very deep effect.

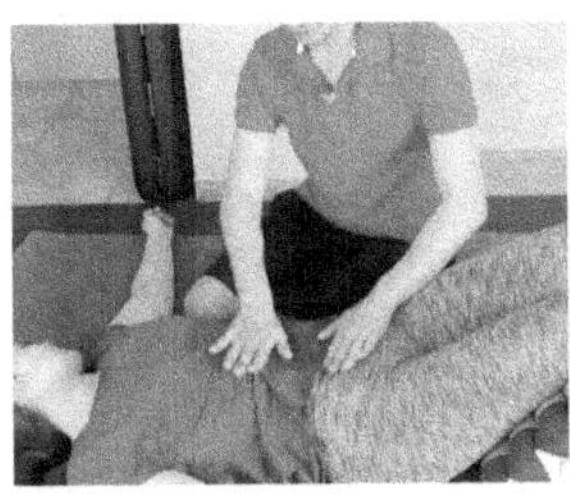

8-Circular friction.

Finish with a clockwise circular rub. Feel free to spend some time with the friction or with the imposition of hands on the area to relax.

---

1. As can be seen, here the kidneys share the emotions of fear and sadness. Source: Nephyr Jackobsen.

CHAPTER 13
SIMPLIFIED THAI ACUPRESSURE

Now I will tell you something that may be very obvious, but that I didn't know when I started Thai massage: not all thumb pressure counts as acupressure.

In Thai massage we constantly use thumb pressure, but this pressure, although it has its therapeutic justification, is not acupressure.

Generally speaking, the aim of this pressure is to go deeper into the body and thus reach deep muscles, arteries, veins and tendons, which are very important structures for movement (of blood and the body).

What Thai acupressure seeks, through specific protocols, is the treatment of certain types of ailments.

If you want to get into this, I recommend the book "Thai Accupressure for Orthopedic Disorders" by Noam Tyroler, with whom I had the privilege of learning firsthand.

Below I will show you two simplified protocols, one for lower back pain and one for neck pain. If you combine these techniques with massage and stretching, you will notice very good results even though it is not a formal acupressure protocol, which is usually more complex and with more points.

There are several ways to stimulate the points, I recommend deep pressure, count 5-10 seconds and change.

SIMPLIFIED ACUPRESSURE FOR LUMBAGO:

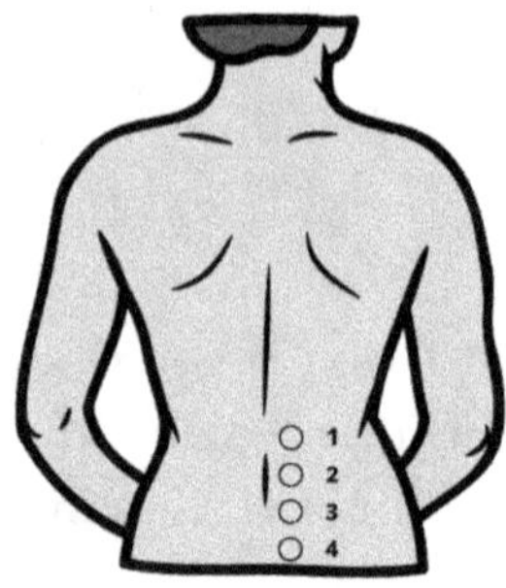

1-POINTS for lower back pain 1.

If the pain is on one side of the back, use these four points. Point 1 is found by locating the floating rib, from where you mark an imaginary line towards the spine, and pressing on line 1, between the vertebra and the paravertebral muscle. Point 4 is above the sacrum. Points 2 and 3 are in the middle, equidistant from points 1 and 4. You can press with your thumbs together, or with your elbow (more carefully this way).

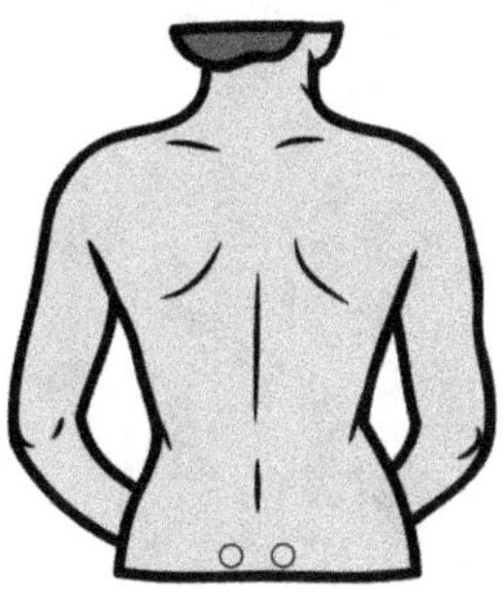

2-POINTS for lower back pain 2.

If the pain is on both sides of the back, press point 4 bilaterally. Remember that this point is above the edge of the sacrum (not over the sacrum).

SIMPLIFIED THAI ACUPRESSURE for neck pain:

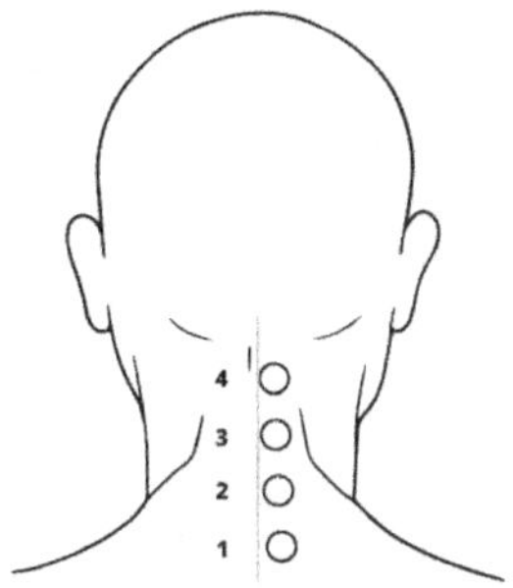

1-POINTS FOR NECK PAIN.

Point 1 is next to C7, where the neck will begin. Point 4 is below the occipital, the skull. Points 2 and 3 are in the middle. Work on the side that hurts, next to the spine.

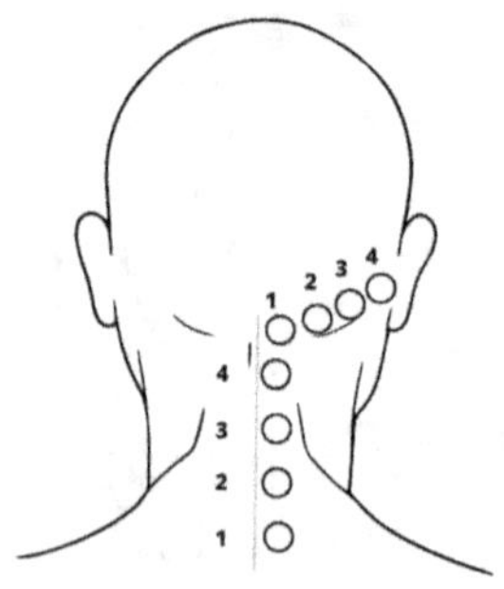

2-Points for treating headaches.

Many times neck pain or discomfort is accompanied by headache, heaviness and/or dizziness. In this case, add the four points above. The first is above cervical point 4, but on the occipital. One finger lengh further towards the ear is point 2, another finger further towards the ear is point 3, and finally one finger further away we find point 4, which would be more or less two fingers from the ear on the occipital. These points, being on the bone, are sensitive so be careful. The pressure you apply is one that the client can withstand.

In each case you can either exert simple pressure, i.e. sustained pressure for 5-10 seconds and exit, or apply circular pressure.

PART III

FREQUENTLY ASKED QUESTIONS AND OTHER ISSUES

In this part, I have included some common questions that people ask me on a regular basis about topics that have to do with the practice of massaging. They will help you understand how to take care of yourself and to recognize the effects that can be observed during work.

CHAPTER 14
FAQ

1 **-How do I know if the type of pressure is the right one?**

Acquiring the right touch is a process that takes time and practice. What you should do to make sure you are doing it right is to practice a lot, preferably with different body types and constantly ask for feedback. It is also a good idea to massage each person several times; once a week would be ideal. That way, not only will you be able to see the immediate effects and sensations you produce, but you will learn to modulate the pressure over time and see better results as well.

2-WHAT ARE THE BENEFITS?

The answer is: it depends. The benefits of a Thai massage do not depend on the technique alone, but on the knowledge and skill of the therapist. If you are at a beginner level, massage will serve to relieve muscle tension and treat states of anxiety and stress very effectively. At more advanced levels it can be used to treat tendinitis, stiffness, headaches, constipation, insomnia, and digestive problems, among others.

3-WITH WHOM CAN **it be performed?**

Again, everything will depend on the experience and skills of the therapist. In therapeutic Thai massage, we can perform it on anyone as long as we know how to work with that particular case. Just as in a yoga class, the postures that are beneficial for some people can be harmful to others. In therapeutic Thai massage we must know how to choose which maneuvers will be most appropriate for each person. What I advise you to do is to practice the protocol of this book with people suffering from common pathologies such as those mentioned in the previous section.

4-I AM TOO OLD / **young / fat / skinny / stiff, will I be able to do Thai massage?**

I have been teaching Thai massage since 2010. Since then hundreds of people have attended my classes. Many of them did not have the ideal qualities for this type of work, nor did they have a special gift. In fact, many of them were suffering from all kinds of difficulties, from stiffness and lack of coordination, to obesity and considerable neurological problems. In all these cases I have seen progress, often spectacular, and they ended up with a better performance than others who had greater ease. What was it that allowed them to excel? The desire to get ahead, the determination to learn something they enjoyed even though it was difficult, the tenacity and willingness to practice over and over again until they got there. So, if you are paying attention to your difficulties and you are unsure whether you can do it or not,

I would tell you to forget about it and follow your heart. One of the most important conditions is the desire to become a Thai therapist.

5-You say that massage helps to balance energy How is this done?

To understand this you need a more advanced knowledge of the technique and the theory of the 4 elements, but I will try to explain it with two simple examples.

Each element has to do with some aspect of our physique, some aspect of our personality, such as the element Lom or Wind, that has to do with movement. When a person has muscle tension, it is a wind problem because the tension impedes the normal movement of the blood and the normal movement of the joint. So when you do compressions and acupressure to relieve tension, you are balancing the energy because you are restoring movement, you are releasing the Lom in the body. When a person suffers from stress, we could say that they suffer from a Lom blockage in the head (because they can't stop thinking, they can't relax). So in that case what we should do is unblock that energy and bring it to their feet, because their feet will send that excess energy to the Earth. The way to do this is to work from top to bottom.

6-What do I need to get started?

What you need is something that allows the client to lie on the floor. It can be a mat, preferably the size of a double bed, 5 cm high and 5 kilos of resistance. These are the optimal characteristics for working on a mat. You can also use yoga mats and blankets. In this case I recommend using at least 3 mats, preferably 5 (three in a row and then one above and one below), and 2 to 5 blankets on top. The most recommended option, if it is within your possibilities, is to get a cotton futon. The optimal size is 1.40 x 2.00. To me they're the best surface for this type of work. Sometimes you can find them on Amazon.com. The good thing about this futon is that it weighs little (about 7 kilos) and it is trans-portable, so you can roll it up and take it everywhere. It is very comfortable (I have even used it to sleep for quite some time). I would also recommend having at least two or three cushions.

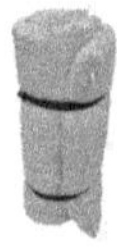

CHAPTER 15
WHAT TO DO IF YOU GET KNEE PAIN

The reason for taking care of your knees, especially when doing Thai massages, is obvious: we spend almost all of our time on the floor. This makes it extremely important that you are aware of any discomfort or pain, as moving on the floor can become uncomfortable if your knees are not in good condition.

The most common reasons why your knees may bother you are:

-Because you are a beginner and you're not used to it. Don't worry, human beings have an amazing capacity for adaptation, you will have to cultivate patience.

-Because you have had a trauma or overexertion.

-Because your joints are a bit worn out. In either case, the best thing to do is not to despair, be patient, and take action so that your own body accelerates the recovery process.

How to relieve knee pain

Are you familiar with harpagofito? It is a root native to southern and southeastern Africa with analgesic and anti-inflammatory properties. It is also known as the "devil's claw". There are several forms of use: oil, ointment, infusion or pills. For convenience, I have tried the pills with considerable success. There are several brands, some of which are even combined with willow extract to enhance the analgesic effect. One to three pills are taken after each meal. In addition to taking the pills and rubbing the oil on yourself, you can make poultice.

How to make a poultice of Devil's Claw

To do this you must make a strong infusion with the root of the devil's claw, boiling for ten minutes one part root to three parts water (preferably mineral). Then you must strain, and with the resulting water (warm) you have to add red clay to make a paste dense enough so that you can apply it on your skin without problems.

It is important that you do not use metal elements in the preparation of the poultice because it would lose its properties, preferably from a bowl or a plastic or wooden spoon or spatula. Once the poultice is made, generously cover your knees and wrap them with plastic wrap (yes, plastic used in the kitchen). If you have a knee pad that is not too tight, use it to keep the preparation firm. You can go to sleep and leave it to act for about four hours. Keep in mind that you need to repeat this operation every day until the pain subsides. Each case is different, but usually within a couple of days you will begin to notice a difference.

Obviously this is only a recommendation, and if in

doubt you should seek the advice of your personal physician. In recent years I must say that devil's claw has become my favorite ally, and I would recommend any of its forms in the medicine cabinet of any therapist for Thai massage, shiatsu or similar.

CHAPTER 16
OTHER COMMON MASSEUR PROBLEMS AND HOW TO AVOID THEM

Over the years, I have had the most varied experiences with thai massage, but I have also had some "wake-up calls". Healthy eating, calisthenics[1] and meditation have kept me strong and healthy for most of my life. However, whenever I have suffered from any discomfort, I have done my best to identify the source so that I can reduce the chances of a new onset of symptoms. I have grouped the conditions resulting from the practice of Thai massage into three major branches: joint disorders, muscle disorders and energy problems.

Joint disorders

The knees

Since the western world has accustomed us to the use of chairs, most of us are not used to being on the floor for any reason. That is why when you start practicing Thai massage, and depending on your level of flexibility, you may experience swelling and pain in the knees, due to the constant movements and displacements on and around the client. In this case it is advisable to be patient and use the devil's claw[2] (which we have already discussed in the previous chapter). It is important to know that the knees eventually get used to it and get stronger, so this is a temporary discomfort. If you are thinking of starting to practice Thai massage and want to avoid this kind of discomfort, I recommend spending more time on the floor to get used to it.

THE WRIST

Another type of ailment has to do with the wrist. This problem usually appears due to an excess of palmar pressure, lack of habit, and probably also by forcing them to an angle that is not entirely natural. This is a type of injury that must be avoided under all circumstances, as it can cause you to have to stop massaging for a while. The best way to prevent this is to distribute your tools evenly. In each session of the Thai massage you use different parts of the body, including the palms, fingers, elbows, forearms, knees and feet. If you use your whole body, the risk of forcing your wrists too hard will be much lower. As in the case of knees, you can use a devil's claw and poultice.

THE SPINE

Although in Thai massage working from the ground facilitates the use of balanced postures, if you are not very body conscious and have acquired postural vices, you may be prone to performing the maneuvers incorrectly, leading you to arch your spine when you should have it straight. If this happens, you may find that after doing a few massages, you may need to get massaged. Of course, if this becomes a habit, the consequences can be serious. To avoid this you should be aware of your posture, and if possible your teacher is the one who should make sure to correct you and convey to you the importance of a healthy posture. You have to keep your back straight at all times during the massage, but also throughout your day. It is for this reason that in my Thai massage classes I put a lot of emphasis on postural correction. If you are used to keeping your back balanced, every massage you do will keep you in shape.

Muscle disorders

Just as poor posture can lead to a problem in your spine, it can also create tension in your muscles. Avoid lifting your shoulders while doing the massage, they should be down and slightly backwards. Also keep your gaze forward, don't spend too much time looking down, this will avoid the stress on your neck. In the same way, if you do not keep your back straight, you may experience discomfort in the lumbar and/or dorsal area. The same is true for the lower back.

Other parts of the body that can accumulate tension are the legs and buttocks. There are some postures that may require some leg strength, depending on the differences in physique and weight between you and your client. The best way to avoid tension after a massage is to get in shape! As I said before, doing Thai massages can keep you in shape, although I prefer the philosophy of training on the side, so that the massage is easy and effortless for me afterwards. I particularly enjoy and recommend calisthenics. A basic but effective workout routine requires only three exercises: squats, push-ups and pull-ups. Do 2 to 4 sets with as many reps as you can, at least three times a week, and you'll be more than ready to keep the massaging from exhausting you. One important thing about these exercises is that you should focus on the perfection of the technique rather than the number of reps. Don't get excited about trying to do 100 push-ups, try to do them slower and with good posture, you will probably do fewer repetitions, but your body will get the benefit of doing it this way.

Energy problems

Finally, another type of disorder you can suffer from has to do with energy use. Many times, our clients come to us not only with problems in their bodies, but also with a level of mental or emotional stress that could affect us if we don't do something about it. What has helped me the most to avoid these types of problems is:

–**Meditation and mindfulness.** Spend a few moments a day concentrating exclusively on your breathing, with no intention of stopping your thoughts, instead just observing them and returning your attention again and again to your breathing. Gradually your mind will become balanced and with it your energy.

–**Seasalt.** Use sea salt in your bath or shower to neutralize toxic energies that may have been passed to you by your client.

–**Stones.** I love stones. To minimize the impact of dense energies, try carrying stones such as shungite, obsidian or onyx with you while you do the massage, or place them in various locations in your cabinet.

–**Recite a mantra while doing the massage.** If you already have some level of practice with Thai massage, and can make your body flow as you go through the work, you can bring your mind to the mental repetition of a mantra. If you don't have one, you can simply recite the sacred syllable "Om", "So Ham", "Jesus" if you are a Christian, or any other sound or mantra that brings you to a special state of consciousness. When the mind concentrates, and especially when it concentrates on a sacred formula, it generates a special vibration that is much stronger than the negative energies of your client.

---

1. A training method in which the body's own weight is used to exercise and strengthen itself. The three best known exercises are pull-ups, squats and push-ups.
2. http://es.wikipedia.org/wiki/Harpagophytum_procumbens

CHAPTER 17
THE EFFECT OF THAI
MASSAGE ON EMOTIONS

It all started the day I had my first client who had a serious emotional breakdown. What to do when, instead of the typical case of muscle tension, you get someone with depression? Will I be able to meet expectations? What techniques should I use? All this was going through my mind in fractions of a second as I filled out the form with my client's data, and asked more questions to delve deeper into the origin of her problem.

Basically it was a state of depression due to the break up with her husband.

None of the Thai massage courses I took, prepared me for such a situation. However, after the first few initial minutes, my doubts were diminishing, and I began to gain confidence in myself and my strategies.

That's how I solved it:

People with anguish and depression are usually cowering forward, with their chests closed, short breaths and gazing at the ground. What does a person with serenity and optimism look like? Quite the opposite, right? Head erect, shoulders relaxed and back, gaze forward, deep and slow breathing. So I set out to "fix" the client's posture so that she would feel like a winner.

Here are some of the manipulations that I recommend focusing on in such cases:

-Scalp and face massage. For relaxation.

-Chest massage (upper pectoral and sternum), to promote deep breathing. Keep in mind that this area is close to the heart, which in Thai medicine is related to joy.

-Palm presses on the shoulders to open the chest and correct posture. Again, opening the chest is essential so that the person can "open up" emotionally again. The closed posture means that there is a protective armor that the person creates to protect him/herself from something that is harming him/herself or he/she thinks is harming him/her.

-Head stretches, so that the head is upright again and helps restore confidence.

-Abdominal massage, we have already seen how it balances the energy of the 4 elements and the relationship between organs and emotions.

-Finally, a lot of palmar pressure and acupressure on the back, especially at the level of the shoulder blades, that is, at the level of the heart. I usually do a Thai massage with the feet and a traction that unblocks the vertebrae at that height. Although the latter is a more advanced technique, simply by doing alternate and simultaneous palm presses you can help to rebalance your client's posture and restore his mood, as shown in the protocol.

The results you can see

Sometimes the changes can be subtle, sometimes dramatic. The cases I will refer to are real, I will just change the names of my clients to preserve their identity.

Julia was a woman of robust physical build, had two small children, and had a lot of problems with her partner and family. This caused her to express herself with a singular verbosity, even several minutes into the message. What I did was simply allow my client to express herself, and work on emphasizing the maneuvers I mentioned above. The result: she gradually fell asleep, and after 15 minutes she ceased all conversation and let herself relax. At the end of the session she was a completely different person, which was evident in her facial expression, her tone of voice and the quality of her words.

Sergio was a strong, yet rigid man. He shied away from talking about matters of the heart or expressing his emotions. He came to the consultation because of back pain, and after only the first session, he not only relieved his physical pain, but also began to express his feelings and reflect on certain behaviors that had led him to be alone. He felt more relieved and was able to heal an emotional wound he had with a former partner.

Eugenia was going through a bad time in her life; she was alone, she had a child, and resources were not abundant. When she released the dorsal area, she immediately started crying, which then gave way to a feeling of relief, "as if I had freed myself from a very big burden," was what she said at the end of the session.

Focus on what is most important

These are just a few cases, but I hope they are compelling enough to make you realize the importance of attending to what is happening to the client on an emotional level.

A person may come to you for typical back pain, but it is

your duty to find out what else is behind that physical pain and target that as well whenever possible.

The client may not know that you can do anything to ease his or her pain from being abandoned, mistreated or misloved, but now you know you can, and you can do it with these simple tips.

CHAPTER 18
THE EFFECT OF MASSAGE ON
THE THERAPIST

Everyone talks about the effects of massage on the client, but we, the therapists, have to be taken into account with equal importance. Which is why in this section I want to talk to you about the effects of Thai massage on you, the therapist.

One of the tools used in Thai massage is passive yoga or assisted stretching. Now, you are probably familiar with the benefits of yoga practice, but can assisted postures benefit the therapist?

Anyone could infer that such bodywork would cause intense physical and energetic wear and tear, and even postural and muscular problems. But this does not necessarily have to be the case.

Thai massage consists of a set of different techniques: stretching, bending, palm presses, finger presses, forearm, elbow and foot presses. With the whole body, the level of wear and tear may be less than a normal massage on a massage table. I say "may" because everything will depend on the techniques chosen by the therapist, and the constitution of the client.

When you have a certain level of mastery of the technique, body awareness and breathing are elements that are put into practice automatically, so that working on the client not only works for the restoration of the health of the recipient but represents respiratory gymnastics, complete body work, and even meditation in motion for the therapist.

Another quality of the technique results from the possibility of using one's own body weight, and this is achieved through a good knowledge of body mechanics. This means that when we work with this intention, our body's awareness increases, and we learn to use it better; we can generate a lot of pressure with the least effort. With this knowledge, the bodywork becomes simpler, and lighter.

Another issue is that of rhythm. I like to compare massage to music. In a massage there must be harmony, balance, and a beat. I must admit that this is not part of the traditional massage, at least not that I know of. Even so, for me it is important. A massage with a good cadence makes the receiver feel better, while the therapist, if he or she can master the movements and changes of posture, can feel them flowing, and dance around the client. It takes some time to learn how to do it when you are a novice, but it is worth the effort. Cadence is a good ingredient in relaxing the client, a fast and disorderly pressure frequency is not the same as a slow and rhythmic one. From the former we can expect more confusion about the stimuli in the client, while in the latter we are more likely to achieve a relaxed state of consciousness, with more receptivity to the treatment and better results.

There is also the issue of breathing. The therapist should maintain a slow and calm breathing throughout the session; this type of breathing promotes a state of inner peace and tranquility, which is then transmitted to the receiver.

Let's not forget that through massage we not only transmit pressure, friction, percussion and other types of physical stimulation, but we also transmit our own mental state, our energy, so the therapist is the first one who should be able to relieve stress, and a good way to do this is through breath control.

After one hour (or as long as the session you work on lasts) maintaining a conscious and controlled breathing, the effect on the therapist is a deep state of serenity.

Finally, there is the issue of consciousness.

The state of consciousness of the therapist when giving a massage is of great importance. A mind focused on service and humility, a humanitarian feeling, will give the therapist the opportunity to grow personally and spiritually.

In short, performing a complete Thai massage treatment translates into gentle gymnastics for the practitioner, as it tones your muscles and relaxes your mental state. The sensation of giving a Thai massage would be similar to that of taking a yoga, tai chi or similar class.

Mastering the technique means, in my humble opinion, not only acquiring the ability to understand and attend to the particular needs of each client, but in promoting and accelerating the healing processes in others, and at the same time, in oneself.

CHAPTER 19
NOW WHAT?

I congratulate you, the first step is always the hardest and you have just taken it.

Now a few final recommendations so that you can get the most out of your experience:

Practice

Many of the doubts that arise from this book will be solved with practice.

Rewrite

I recommend that you get a notebook and describe in your own words each maneuver, this will help you remember and understand them better.

Visualize

Elite athletes use this technique a lot, where they imagine themselves doing the training as if they were doing it for real. Several studies have shown that it actually helps to improve performance. To help you with this, I have created a video version of the protocol in this book, you can get it at https://learnthaimassage.net/videoguide or by scanning the QR code below.

CONNECT AND MOVE FORWARD

If you liked this book and you are interested in expanding your knowledge, having a deeper impact with your therapies and having a lot of new tools at your disposal, I recommend you to visit my gallery of in-person and online courses at shivathai.net.

FOR ANY QUESTIONS contact me at contacto@shivathai.net, or via WhatsApp at +34-644-025-389.

PART IV

APPENDIX

Here I am going to present you with a series of topics related to the life of a massage therapist. It includes experiences and lessons that have to do with personal, professional, spiritual and economic aspects. I think all of this is relevant and interesting, because your growth as a therapist will be determined in large part by your growth as a person.

CHAPTER 20
THREE LIMITING BELIEFS TO AVOID AS A MASSAGE THERAPIST

I had started taking massage courses for pure pleasure, and up to that point the word "work" meant to me simply a means to make a living, not something I could enjoy.

The thing is that that first month that I started my professional practice as a masseuse, I still had my office job and was fully dependent on that salary. It was a great surprise when I realized, at the end of the month, that I had some extra money that I had no idea about, because it was the first time I was earning money as a masseuse!

For the first time in my life, I had generated income doing something I deeply loved, what a phenomenal feeling!

The problem is that it took me many years to be able to devote myself completely to the activity, because I needed the resources that my office job gave me.

Now that I look back, I can recognize certain mental patterns that limited me and kept me from achieving my goals.

Belief N°1: "People don't have money to get massages because of the crisis".

In every financial crisis in history there have been people who have managed to grow financially despite the circumstances. So, if you are going to make a living from your massage, why not target an audience that wants and can afford to pay for your services?

When I go out on the street I still see people spending money on clothes, jewelry, alcohol, junk food, and going to the bar - how can there not be money for a good massage?

The crisis may be working in our favor. As many people are more and more stressed by this situation, more and more people will turn to a natural solution that makes them feel good about where they are and what they have. And guess what, the massage meets that requirement!

The thing is simple: if you think the crisis will stop you from getting clients, that's what will happen. So look around you and instead of looking at the news about pay cuts and tax hikes, look at the people who are still growing, you can be one of them easing the pain of the hordes of stressed out people!

Belief #2: "People don't pay for massages because it is a luxury item".

This is another chip that I had implanted in my brain and that meant that, despite being very good at doing massages, I could not get the clients I needed.

The point here is to know how to educate our clients and prospects and make them see the value of a healthy and natural life.

If we manage to make them see that their massage is not

an expense or a whim but something that will make them feel strong and alive, that will increase their capacity to enjoy life, then our work will be seen as an investment.

Logically this can be directly linked to your ability to achieve results. You have to be good enough to keep most of your clients satisfied.

Belief #3: "If I'm good, the customers will come to me on their own".

Wrong! I believe without a doubt that if I had detected this pattern earlier, I would now have amassed a considerable fortune.

I will not argue that one should concentrate on improving technique and learning other styles of massage, but that is not the only requirement for success as a massage therapist.

If you want to make a living from massage or improve your income as a massage therapist, you must dedicate some of your time, effort and money to learning how to market yourself. Yes, I'm talking about marketing!

I know that many here will disagree, get angry and think that I am deviating from the true mission of the therapist. But let me tell you one thing: how many people would you help if no one knew you and you didn't know how to reach your audience?

You will probably end up massaging your family and friends (that's all well and good, of course, but you can't make a living at it). With a little luck and time, you can build up a small portfolio of clients thanks to referrals from your acquaintances. But with today's competition and the speed at which the market moves, do you think a small handful of acquaintances will be enough?

My best advice is to spend some of your time studying marketing. You must learn how to reach your potential audience and transform them into customers.

There are also a number of other skills that will be useful to you, for example, knowing how to manage your time, how to manage your money, how to have a successful mindset, how to have an internet presence, and a long list of other skills.

It is true, there is a lot to study, and a lot to work on. However, no one said it would be easy. You can also enjoy, learn, and grow as a therapist and entrepreneur.

In my particular case, since I dedicate part of my time to study marketing in addition to everything related to my profession as a massage therapist, I have managed to be recognized as an authority in my field. And with this, not only can I help more people and make a positive impact in their lives, I can also generate income that allows me to live decently and continue investing in my education and personal growth. If you need help with this, consult me for mentoring sessions.

CHAPTER 21
THAI MASSAGE AS A
SACRED PRACTICE

One of my teachers, Yogi Sarveshwarananda Giri, once told me the story of Brother Lorenzo.

Brother Lawrence was born in France in the 17th century. He lived an ordinary life until the beginning of his adulthood, when he decided to enter a monastery, not knowing quite what to do with his life.

Simply put, Brother Lawrence adopted the practice of chatting with God at every moment, and dedicating each of his actions to Him.

Having been put in charge of the kitchen chores, and without this being his favorite activity (it is said that in fact he rather disliked it), he got into the habit of giving himself to his duties for the love of God. So, for each task he would look up to heaven and say: "God, now I will wash your dishes," or "God, now I will sweep your children's kitchen."

The point is that Brother Lawrence became a saint, but little is known in the West about this character, perhaps because he himself fled from recognition claiming that "external entertainments spoil everything".

Already at the end of his life, he confessed that in his

eagerness to know and perceive the essence of God, he had tried various methods, and that nothing had given him more results than to offer each of his acts with love. His secret lay in the fact that his worldly activities and his moments of prayer were no different. Such was his love and concentration, that not even the coarsest tasks distracted him from the presence of the Divine.

How does Brother Lorenzo's life relate to Thai massage?

What remains for me as a lesson from the life of this great soul, is that if an activity as common as sweeping or washing dishes can lead us to have a personal experience with God, Thai massage, as a sacred healing activity also can do that.

The key is then, to offer that service that we are about to give to our client, to God, under any of his forms or names. Be it Yahweh, Allah, Buddha, Krishna, or Shiva, my suggestion is that you offer that massage session to the idea of God that is most familiar to you according to your culture or inclination. And if you do not have a defined belief, I suggest that when you make the initial greeting before the massage, close your eyes and project into your mind a bright light, or make the effort to bring a sense of peace and harmony to your heart. Or a value that you fervently believe in, such as justice, brotherhood, or compassion.

Another way of working to achieve this state could be to repeat a mantra over and over with the rhythmic sequence of palm and finger presses. I have put it into practice in the following way: mentally repeating the first syllable of the mantra, and then exhaling the second. For example, I repeat "Shivo" on the inhale, and "ham" on the exhale (this mantra means "I am Shiva").

You can do the same with any other mantra, be it the OM-MANI-PADME-HUM of the Buddhists, the OM-

SHANTI, mantra for peace, or the repeating of the name Jesus. The idea is that you coordinate the syllables with the breath and the pressures, and that you choose the name or mantra that most represents you or the one assigned to you by your teacher.

I can assure you that it is a very powerful practice that will expand your consciousness, while achieving a better connection with the person receiving the massage, in addition to improving the quality of the treatment. Don't forget that we are channels of everything that happens inside us when we touch someone, so if you reach a state of peace and serenity during the session, you will transmit the same to your client.

By setting your intention to take the massage as a sacred practice, and that message makes a difference for you and your client, you succeed in transforming your treatment into a spiritual experience. Dedicate the message to God, to a saint you revere (as a Thai therapist you might choose Shivago), or to your teacher. Incorporate a mantra or the name of the Divine that is most familiar to you, and make the Thai massage session a true meditative dance that leads you to understanding the Absolute and union with the Eternal.

CHAPTER 22
HOW TO IMPROVE YOUR JOB OPPORTUNITIES WITH THAI MASSAGE

Alfons Cornella, in his book Visionomics, states that "in an industrial society, workers' wages are based on the fulfillment of a scheduled time period." In service-centered societies, a large portion of wages depend on the objectives achieved. In contrast, the worker of the 21st century will receive a large part of his or her salary for having differential knowledge.

I think this statement applies perfectly to all fields, including the massage therapy itself. In a market as competitive as this one, a superfluous knowledge of massage techniques will no longer be enough; you will have to research, practice and learn constantly, so that you can show your future employers that you can not only offer better service, but a massage with your own style, where you can give more of yourself, and stand out from the competition.

The best way to learn

That's why in my school I highlight the importance of following to the letter each of the Thai massage routines we teach, and then forget them and create your own protocols based on your experience and intuition. In other words, we give you the rules, and the permission to break them! --

While instead of repeating the same massage routine, you will be creating them from the knowledge you have acquired, you will not only be growing as a therapist, you will also be able to enjoy your work more. And if you enjoy it more, others will perceive it, and you will be providing an added value that not everyone will be able to provide. You increase your chances of success in front of your employers and in front of your clients.

On board for success

This is what happened to me when I went to apply for a job with Steiner, a multinational cruise ship spa services company.

There were about forty or fifty people at the interview. To top it off, we had to come to the front to speak in English in public. Then there was a written evaluation, followed by a massage on makeshift massage tables.

I made a very positive impression on them with a combination of Swedish massage, sports massage, and Thai acupressure with stretching. The result: I was immediately selected and sent to London for special training.

Once working officially for Steiner, on Royal Caribbean's largest cruise ships, I was just another massage therapist on a staff of more than a dozen therapists.

In the spa environment, women tend to be preferred over men, sensuality and softness over therapeutic skill, and (much to my regret) beautiful therapists in their twenties over bald men over thirty.

""I'm fucked," I thought. But I discovered that I could take advantage of my apparent disadvantage. That's where Thai massage helped me bring that differential value that allowed me to stand out and earn a lot of money.

The spa protocol did not allow traditional Thai massage, but said nothing about Thai acupressure or stretching on a massage table. So I began to sell my services by highlighting this difference in relation to the treatments offered by my colleagues.

What happened was that I ended up making as much or more money than my colleagues, who sold their services because they were young and pretty women. I don't want to say that they were only doing well because of that, but it is true that these qualities were a great advantage for them (and a great disadvantage for me).

Advice:

1. If you want to get a job and you are having a hard time, do not give up, instead of despairing, occupy your mind with learning new skills and moving forward. Invest in classroom courses, videos and books -- remember that differential knowledge is what people are looking for these days.

2. Learn therapeutic Thai massage techniques to enhance your resume and your therapeutic skills. If you already know Thai massage, continue learning through other courses/exchanges with colleagues, or opening yourself to other styles to enrich your technique. If you are a beginner, Thai massage will also give you invaluable knowledge about your body, and who knows, maybe even the possibility of changing your life.

3. Don't watch the news about the crisis and unemployment. It will only discourage you from concentrating on your goals and moving forward.

CHAPTER 23

HOW MUCH CAN YOU EARN DOING MASSAGE?

The first thing you should know before you read on is: don't do it for the money. This profession, like any other, has its ups and downs, its pros and cons, and when faced with challenges, if you only do it for the money, you will have a very bad time and you simply won't be able to stand it. Having made this clarification, and knowing that you love massaging and helping others, let's analyze some key points:

Having a job

Importantly, if you are looking for a job at a massage center or spa, your earnings will be much lower than what you can get working on your own. Of course, as you can imagine, the advantage of working for someone else is that you can concentrate on your treatments, and you enjoy a certain "stability", in the sense that while you work, you will receive your salary, which is a good thing. Logically the ceiling of what you can earn is going to be determined by the company you work for and the amount of hours you work.

Let's say you work 30 - 40 hours a week, your salary could be around €1,000 - €1,500, (remember, it will always depend on the company, where it is located, and the working conditions they offer).

When I worked for Steiner as a spa therapist on cruise ships, I had no salary; what I earned came from commissions for services and sales of spa products on the one hand, and tips from clients on the other. Despite the fact that this is a job, here we are talking about a different world. Why? Well, because when you work for this company, your earnings will be determined by the volume of public (and the socioeconomic level) that the spa has, and this will depend on the cruise line that you are sent to and the route it takes. Thus, it is not the same to be sent to a new cruise ship than to an older one, it is not the same to be sent to a ship with a 7-day tour of the best beaches in the Caribbean, than to one that makes three ports that are not very crowded, or a tour around the world. For each one, you will earn differently depending on the type of client and the consumption habits of the client. I won't go into detail here about the different variables, but I can tell you that, on average, I earned between $400 and $600 a week in tips plus my commissions (this was in 2009). Keep in mind that not every week and month was the same, and that the work required very long and strenuous days, but it still worked out well for me.

Becoming an entrepreneur

Okay, here we also have to consider different things like:

-How much would you charge? The cheaper you charge, the more it will cost you to have a decent income at the end of the month. Also, the more you can charge, the more you can take care of yourself, invest in your education and infrastructure to provide better services, and so on. There is also a question of self-esteem here: how much do you value your work? If you value it little, you can't expect others to.

Do you have that experience and self-confidence? This is one of the most important variables, the more experience you have, the better you will get and the more results you will be able to achieve, ergo, you will be able to charge more. At the same time, the more confidence you have, the easier it will be to add value to your services. Important: don't wait until you have confidence in yourself to have experience (i.e. get to work with clients), go out and have experience, and you will see how you gain confidence.

-What audience will you target? Pure logic, if your audience can't afford the value of your therapies, don't lower the prices, target another audience!

-Where will you work? This is related to the above, if you see that a place you want to work does not have an audience open to the type of services you want to provide, then go find that audience elsewhere.

-Do you have an effective customer acquisition strategy? It is no longer enough to go out to mailboxes or paste flyers on lampposts, you have to learn to work with other marketing channels, including online marketing.

-How many hours do you plan to dedicate to it? If your financial goals are not very ambitious, you could easily dedicate yourself part-time, that is, between one and three hours a day.

-How much competition do you have? I really didn't know whether to include this variable, because although it does have to do with what you can charge or not, it is also true that if you get very good and have a good marketing strategy, people will prefer you over others, regardless of the price. Remember this: at the level of excellence there is no competition, become extremely good, become unique, and your competition will be irrelevant.

Let's talk about pricing

My intention in this book is not to teach you about pricing, but what I can tell you is this: the price has nothing to do with the technique or how it is used. I am often asked, "How much can I charge for a Thai massage?" What happens is that you cannot offer a price for that type of technique, because the price is the most subjective thing there is. Think about it, there is no rule that establishes how much you can charge, so basically you could charge from €0 to... what do you think? €50? €100? €200? If I told you €400, would you believe me? Personally, when I worked at the Royal Caribbean spas, I got to do a treatment worth over $300 (mind you, that's what the company charged). Okay Cesar, but there is still €150 missing. All right, well, I tell you that I once met a shiatsu master who charged $250 per half hour treatment, that is about $500 per hour, and this was in 2006 money and in Argentina! Did people pay him? Of course they did! He was a renowned figure with a great trajectory, so people happily paid him. I know, at this point you are probably thinking that you are not exactly a prominent figure in the massage world, and that if tomorrow you were to put your sessions at €500 per hour your place would be more deserted than the Sahara.

Don't worry, you don't need to be famous or to charge a premium, let's do some simple math. Let's say you charge €50 an hour per session, and you only do two massages a day from Monday to Friday, and at the end of the month it would be €2,000. Okay, we have to take out the self-employed fee, vats and so on, but it is still good money to work only two hours a day. Now imagine that instead of two massages a day, you do four, and that you also work on Saturdays, in which case at the end of the month you would have disbursed €4800. One last case scenario. Masseuse X, living in Girona, Spain, earns €50 and works 7 hours a day, 4 in the morning and 3 in the afternoon, from Monday to Friday. That translates into 140 massages per month, and a total of €7,000. I know it all sounds very nice and that at the end of the day they are just numbers and estimates, but believe me, they are achievable figures, I know several professionals who earn €2,000, €3,000, €5,000, and even €9,000 or €10,000 per month. I'm not going to fool you, these people make a good living, but they work hard, they take care of their clients and their business, they have a good marketing strategy, and they are constantly learning and investing to improve their skills. While it is also true that these results are not achieved overnight, having ambition is fine - but you have to dedicate time, perseverance, and be willing to make mistakes and learn all the nuances of massaging as a business.

Conclusion

What I would like you to take away from this chapter is this exercise:

-Tally up all the expenses you have in your life per month.

-Think about the number, the exact figure you would like to earn per month.

-Calculate the price you will charge and the number of sessions you would have to do to reach that goal.

-Do something every day to promote yourself and write down in a spreadsheet or notebook how many massages you do per week and what you are earning (don't forget to subtract expenses!).

-Keep a portion of everything you earn to continue investing in improving your skills.

-Analyze the results at least once a month, and move on.

Also, don't be afraid to think about a high figure, maybe it will take you more time, maybe your plan will not turn out as you expected, but if you put in enough effort, dedicate time, lose the fear of making mistakes, and have patience, I assure you that inexorably you will be able to earn what you want doing massage sessions.

CHAPTER 24
HOW I HELPED MY FATHER RECOVER FROM A STROKE WITH THAI MASSAGE

I discovered my vocation with massages almost by chance. Massage therapy gave me a different way to express myself, to help people, to contribute to the world, and as it turned out, to make a living. But if there's one thing I didn't expect, it was this strange and wonderful feeling of communicating on a much deeper level with the people I loved.

History repeated itself with a different ending

My father grew up in a family of nine siblings in rural Paraguay. Things were going well until my grandfather passed away when my father was 6 years old. From then on, the family economy collapsed, forcing my father and his siblings to go through all kinds of hardships to survive. Perhaps it was these kinds of things that we common mortals interpret as "misfortunes" that made my father a fighter.

At the age of 37, when I was 6, he had to have an operation on his head to unblock an artery partially plugged with fat. "It's just preventive," said the doctors. We had a Cesarito Sandoval for almost twenty more years, without too many complications, until one day what we all feared, was about to happen.

I was returning from my summer vacation, and as soon as I walked through the door of my house I found out that my father had suffered a stroke and was hospitalized. As soon as I arrived, I took off my bags and went to the hospital. The outlook was not very encouraging, but everyone in the family was hopeful that he would survive, once again.

Things were not easy and, as a consequence of the incident, my father was left without mobility from the neck down, and he had also lost mobility in his facial muscles, so, although fully conscious, he could not articulate words well, so we had to make an effort to understand him and communicate with him.

Now what?

This was the situational picture; the question was what to do. As a massage therapist, I had faith that the skills I had acquired while working on Swedish and Thai massage would pay off. No academy had prepared me to deal with such a complicated client, so I brought out some common sense and a lot of faith in God.

This is what I did

My father was literally lying motionless in bed, so I started giving him very gentle Swedish massage sessions right there. I started with short 30-minute sessions, and each day I increased the duration by a few minutes.

Within two weeks a miracle happened: my father was able to get out of bed! Not only that, but his facial muscles seemed to be recovering as well, and so was his ability to communicate verbally.

My father was a sheet metal worker in the car industry

all his life, so the normal thing for him was to have a car and drive, so it was almost like another part of his body. So when he told us one day, "I'll drive again,". No one wanted to convey to him the implausibility of his statement.

Thai massage for rehabilitation

When Papa Cesar managed to start moving, I was encouraged to take him to the futon (at that time my futon was a couple of old quilts covered with a sheet), and to give him his first Thai massage sessions.

Those first sessions were extremely basic, like the ones I teach in this book: just a few palm presses on the whole body, and some mobilization.

Over time I added more complex maneuvers, and spaced out the sessions a bit. I even had the luxury of performing maneuvers considered contraindicated for cardiac, diabetic and hypertensive people like my father. This validates my idea that sometimes it's not so important what you do, but how you do it.

I realized that book prescriptions are just that, book prescriptions, they serve to guide the therapist, who must adjust the rules to the particular situation. And in this case, I felt that I could do the pulse stop, I could do slightly stronger pressures, and also some inverted postures[1] (all contraindicated for a case like my father's).

In his particular case it was a question of duration and intensity. Once in the middle of the massage, I felt a certainty that on that occasion, everything was going to work well -- I just had to execute the slower, gentler manipulations.

The point is that after about six months, my father regained enough mobility to lead a normal life. He could no longer exert himself and was forced to stay away from strong emotions, but he was able to continue taking Thai massage sessions, and also, a few months later, he managed to drive again.

Warning

First of all, I want to warn you that my intention is not to encourage you to go against what the books say and ignore the contraindications. Contraindications are useful, they are a guide, and you should pay attention to them to avoid causing harm.

My intention is to point out that there are certain situations in which the only way to be effective is to break the rules. But to do this you have to have a lot of experience, common sense, and above all, a strong sense of responsibility. One of the reasons Thai massage, as I did it, worked despite the precarious state my father was in, was because I had a strong emotional connection with him. This is not to say that an emotional connection is necessary, but it can help.

Thai massage can be used to help people with serious disorders, but to do it well, you must inform yourself about your client's illness, in all possible ways. Your contribution, as in my case, will be a helpful complement to traditional treatments. In cases like these, rather than substituting one medicine for another, we should talk about collaborating, beyond our opinions and favoritism towards natural therapies.

---

1. These are the positions at which we lift the recipient's legs above his body.

CHAPTER 25
LIFE LESSONS LEARNED THROUGH THAI MASSAGE

In 2003, when I took my first Thai massage class, I thought I was learning an interesting ethnic, traditional and therapeutic technique. With a little time and practice I realized that this was not only so, there was more valuable and deeper learning to be gained from the technique. Here I will summarize some of those lessons.

1-Everyone and everything is your teacher

I have learned that one cannot always count on a great teacher, but at all times one has the opportunity to become a great apprentice. You can learn by attending classes, giving massages, receiving them -- you can learn from an experience that has served you, and from one that has not. Because opportunities to learn are everywhere, one must learn how to identify them.

When I had the opportunity to live in Thailand, back in 2009, I had a lot of massage treatments. And, as expected, not all of the sessions were good. Still, I learned a lot, both from experiences that exceeded my expectations and those that did not.

2-We are a small piece of a large gear...

When we start working, we want all of our clients to get better no matter what situation they are in. In reality, if the person who comes to your office does not improve, it does not necessarily mean that you are doing something wrong. Each individual is like a complex and complete universe in itself; we are just a small piece that makes some adjustments to the big machinery that is the client's life. This complexity means that we must adopt a position of humility, both in the success and failure of our mission of helping our clients improve their health and wellbeing. We are instruments of something bigger than ourselves.

3-Working towards caring for others implies taking better care of yourself.

Our bodies, minds and energy are the vehicles that allow us to work and perform. In the field of massage therapy, this law is fulfilled without any mercy, and those who do not take it seriously, those who do not take care of themselves, often pay the price of injuries that harm their performance and even force them to abandon the profession.

So, if you want to enjoy this profession, you must take care of yourself. Do research on natural foods and on methods of self-cleansing and purification, meditate, exercise regularly, and eliminate any vices that are intoxicating you. This means that you will not only be able to work smoothly, but you will also feel better overall and serve as an example and motivation for your clients.

4-It is good to be pragmatic, but it is also necessary to pay attention to what you feel.

When I set out to learn Thai massage, I had little idea how all this knowledge would serve me (it was a time when I was not planning to become a professional and I was studying English translation at university). Reason told me that it would be very difficult to capitalize on all that I was willing to invest in my training. I decided to listen to my intuition, and that radically changed my life forever. It is not that this is going to happen to everyone, nor that the reasoning is useless, I am simply testifying to what happened in my particular case. Following my heart led me to meet places and people that I would never have imagined in life. Moral reasoning is useful, but sometimes intuition can help break down the barrier to what you conceive to be impossible.

The same is true in the field of therapy. When you have acquired a certain knowledge of the why of each maneuver, of the theory behind the massage, your technical quality can be very good. Your reason can guide you because you know you can trust it. However, the use of intuition can take you much further.

Thai massage and acupressure master Noam Tyroler, whom I deeply admire, said, "studying acupressure protocols is fine, but when it comes to working with clients, it is better to combine protocols, not follow one specific one."

That is to say that once you have a great knowledge of the protocols, what is more useful is to improvise with a higher level of perception, our hearts, and our sense of what's best in a specific situation.

5-Habit is the important thing

During my first stage of training, I made it a point to never let a week go by without practicing Thai. And it was thanks to this constancy that I came to understand the practice, incorporate it, and achieve a good degree of mastery. I realized that the best results are achieved with small steps on a regular basis, rather than with large, inconsistent steps. With patience, perseverance and discipline you can master any art.

6- And the most important of all...

You never stop learning. Today, having been a trainer for over two decades now, I see that I learn even more, both from my students and from the wonderful experience of interacting with them. Best of all, I will never stop being a student; I will always have lessons to learn from Thai massage, and I'm sure you will too.

ABOUT THE AUTHOR

Cesar Ariel Sandoval was born in Buenos Aires, Argentina, and discovered his vocation as a masseur in 2002, at a time when he was studying at the University of Buenos Aires as a public translator and working as a government employee.

In 2003 he became acquainted with traditional Thai massage and began his journey as a Thai therapist, researching and learning from the different lineages of Thai masters and from different schools around the world.

In 2009 he worked as a spa therapist for Steiner, which led him to work on four ships from Royal Caribbean Cruises, sailing through the Caribbean and several other European and American countries, including the United States.

Between 2009 and 2010 he travels to Southeast Asia and travels to Vietnam, Cambodia, Thailand, Burma and India, where he reinforces everything he learned in previous years and learns new and different styles of massages and other forms of massage therapy.

In 2010 he settled in Barcelona, where he founded Shivathai, a school of traditional Thai massage.

He currently lives in Tarragona, and offers in-person courses in Barcelona, as well as online programs through his website shivathai.net.

ACKNOWLEDGMENTS

I want to thank the people who helped me in one way or another to get this book to see the light of day.

To my friend Javier Ma (founder of ReikiEnTuVida), for his motivation, support and friendship. To Elisabet Ledesma Ramon, for modeling for the majority of the photos and videos that have been posted online. To Federico Nale for the pictures and his friendship.

Also, to the following people who collaborated in the review and promotion: Alberto Martínez Rodríguez, Ana Fernández Rodríguez, Antonio de Jesús Neri Orozco, Carolina San José González de Valladolid, Consuelo Barascan Ayuela, Esther Fortes Fenollos, Eva Caridad Moreno González, Gabriela Miño, José Antonio Carmona Gonzalez, Leire Herce, Lorena Mendo Mier, Pablo Pazos, Puri Duque Duque, Mabel Lao, Mabel López López, Magdalena Mikolaeva, María Isabel Holguín Flores, María del Mar Migueiz Santin, Mayte Mangas, Meritxell Pont Alsina, Noelia Terrón Torres, Silvana Valdés Bravo, y Sandra Alejandra Valverde Parejo.

I also want to thank you for taking the time to read this book. If you have any questions you can write to me at contacto@shivathai.net.

YOU MAY ALSO BE INTERESTED IN

"Medicine Mandalas": Coloring book for adults with self-hypnosis techniques for happiness and wellbeing.

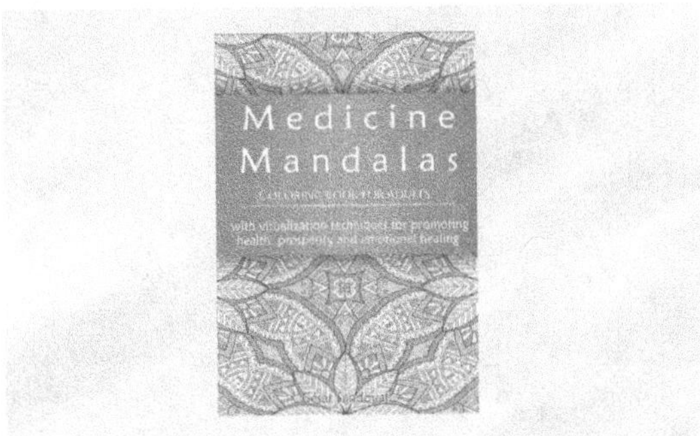

Coming soon "Thai Massage on a Table": thai massage techniques to improve your knowledge and enhance the client experience.

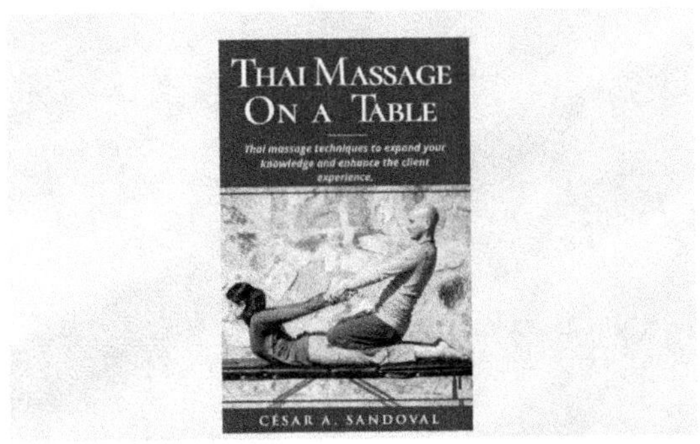